To your Transformation Beautiful One! Mia

TAPPING

TRANSFORM YOUR WORLD

MIA DOUCET

ISBN: 978-0-9959586-2-3

Bankerman Press

To Aria and Piper

May you always be happy.

Contents

Acknowledgments

I AM GRATEFUL TO my wonderful friends and clients whose trust, stories and breakthroughs made this book a possibility.

At the top of the list are the brilliant Jane Girouard and Sneha Radia whose insights helped shape its content and structure.

My thanks to Amelia Does who edited the first iteration of the text and Lisa Bruchac, Janet Christensen, and Lee Johnstone who read and critiqued an early draft.

I am especially grateful to Dr. Eric Robins for agreeing to read the manuscript, then offering to write a Foreword and contributing his medical expertise in a bonus chapter.

I thank Sylvia Hartmann (Positive EFT) and Sandi Radomski, Tom Altaffer and Pamela Altaffer (Ask & Receive) for allowing me to incorporate their methods into the text.

Also deserving of my thanks is my mentor/business coach and friend, John Chancellor, who encouraged me to stop hiding my light and finally release this writing into the world. I am the beneficiary of his potent mind and spirit.

And finally, I want to recognize two creative people who made my book come alive: Ivan Stojić for book layout and cover design, and Anthony O. Yoingco for his genius in translating my stories into charming little pen and charcoal sketches.

FOREWORD

WHAT WAS LIFE changing for me and my practice was when I first discovered EFT back in 1997. At that time, I was actually taking a class to get certified in Roger Callahan's Thought Field Therapy. While I enjoyed that course immensely, I kept thinking to myself, "There are only 14 meridian end points that we are using, why not just tap on all of them each time, rather than having to remember complex algorithms?"

Shortly thereafter, I learned about EFT and have never looked back.

What I liked about EFT was that it was fast enough to use in a busy clinical setting, and allowed us to clear the emotional charge off of past traumas at a deep enough level that physiological shifts occurred, and then the body was able to heal itself.

In addition to shifting physiology, I feel that tapping is also helping to remove energetic blockages in the body. And the science is showing (along with functional MRI scans) that tapping helps to positively influence certain parts of the brain's limbic system that play a role in initiating the stress response.

Even when I didn't have the time to do a full session on a patient, teaching them EFT gave them a powerful tool for daily stress reduction.

Using lots of case studies and metaphors, Mia Doucet has picked up on some of the principles and techniques I have found most useful in my practice.

Some of the overarching principles and components necessary for real and sustained healing that she so beautifully articulates in her book include:

- The understanding that the only thing that's real is now; if we have strong emotions or reactions coming up, and there is actually nothing happening at this moment to affect our safety and well-being, then we are in a hypnotic trance state (and experiencing conditioned neurological responses). A person needs to break free of this trance state in order to heal.

- The need to focus on noticing the raw physical sensations in your body, to be there fully, to not attach meanings or labels to these sensations, to not judge them as good or bad, and to just tap on the awareness of the sensations.

- The fact that, as NLP teaches, there is an underlying structure for most problems. Mia spends ample time explaining how to find the underlying structure of a problem in order to tap on it and release its hold on us.

- The importance of gratitude and focusing on what is working in our lives, as espoused by renowned EFT teacher Silvia Hartmann.

I find this book to be very well written, and I personally resonate with a number of the wonderful stories and metaphors that Mia shares, including many from her own life struggles.

Incorporating the ideas, strategies and methods explained in this book, you may well Transform Your World.

And, if you are a practitioner, you will likely experience a lot more freedom and happiness in both your own and your clients' lives.

Godspeed!

Eric B. Robins, M.D.
Urologist and Mind-Body Healing Specialist
Co-author, "Your Hands Can Heal You"

INTRODUCTION

ALMOST WITHOUT EXCEPTION, the man or woman who contacts me has been attempting without success and for a very long time to create deep positive change in their life.

They tell me they have been tapping on their own or with practitioners for months – and sometimes years, using various energy techniques. What has kept them going is hope, based on the spectacular results promised in tapping summits, teleseminars, webinars and YouTube videos.

That hope has not been fulfilled. And they are tired of dancing around the edges.

IS THIS BOOK FOR YOU?

This book presumes you have previous experience with tapping. It is for you if you have tried tapping along with others, on your own, or with a practitioner and it has not yet transformed your life.

So it is not for the person who is new to the world of meridian tapping. There are many excellent books and videos on the market that would be a better introduction to the method.

It is also not directed to tapping practitioners, although readers of the original manuscript have suggested that practitioners also would get value from the insights and case studies.

One Practitioner's Perspective

This book provides insights and observations based on my own healing journey and working with so many wonderful, committed people over the past eight years.

Other practitioners may or may not agree with them or with my approach. They will have their own stories to tell and their own perfectly valid views based on their own experiences.

I do realize that I may annoy many who have strong loyalties and opinions regarding the virtue of one tapping modality versus another.

My position is that every tapping method has its strengths and is brilliant in its own right.

I heard a respected practitioner say, on a teleseminar, that "tapping takes off the jagged edge." It does do that. Wonderfully.

You can always use tapping to dial down life's everyday tensions and stresses.

But this book assumes that you, the reader, are not just wanting to work on the jagged edges. You want to make over certain parts of your life. When you say tapping doesn't work for you, you mean it hasn't dislodged the deeper issues. It hasn't transformed your life. You are not yet at peace.

THE PROBLEM WITH TAPPING SCRIPTS

I have a bias against canned tapping scripts because they don't fix upon your unique needs. They are too generic to make you happier, richer and more at peace with yourself.

After listening for countless hours, they never worked for me and they haven't worked for the people who seek me out.

The secret to tapping success is not to say the right words. The secret is to access the *origin* of our pain: the invisible, underlying, often unacknowledged emotions that are the *root cause* of our suffering.

When tapping seems not to work it's because we haven't yet got to that root cause.

To be fair, scripts work for some people some of the time. In my experience, they work for people whose issues are not as deep-seated as mine were and yours may be. They work for those whose intrinsic orientation to life is a positive one. (I fondly refer to them as having been born with a "Yes" as opposed to people like me, who were born with a colicky "No.")

They're the lucky ones.

WHAT YOU CAN EXPECT

Part I addresses the issue of WHEN and WHY tapping seems not to work for so many people. It explores 23 reasons – in no particular order – that I have identified in my own life and professional practice that explain why many of us – even trained therapists and practitioners – find it difficult to achieve transformation on our own.

My own story in the first chapter reflects many of the themes that intertwine throughout the chapters in this section: the impact of early childhood events that imprint core beliefs before we have any frame of reference, life themes, repetitive patterns, unconscious programming, trauma and brain shock.

All the examples used to illustrate the 23 reasons are from my files. You will read verbatim excerpts from one-on-one client sessions. Out of respect, I have not included dialogue from any of the more sensitive situations.

With the exception of my one-time assistant Amelia who got a kick out of having her name in this book, all client names are fictitious. For that reason, names appear in quotes the first time they are used.

Part II answers some general questions you may still have about tapping.

In Part III I suggest HOW to unlock the secrets to tapping success if you are attempting personal transformation on your own.

HOW TO GET THE MOST OUT OF THIS BOOK

You could always start by skipping over to the pictures! It's probably a good idea to begin by reading Part I: Reason #1 first. From there, you might skim through the list of 23 reasons for those that resonate with you.

Beyond stories and insights, you will get the greatest value from this book by taking action and following suggested guidelines in Part III.

ONE LAST THING . . .

I want to acknowledge that some people reading this text – particularly those who have had a difficult life – may take exception to my use of humor in some of the following accounts.

To them I want to say that humor that arises naturally out of a situation serves a delightful purpose. Humor is healing.

When we can laugh at something from our past it loses its hold on us. So if a client allows me to reframe a painful thing in a way that they are now able to view it from a comical stance, true healing can take place rapidly.

THE JOY AND THE PASSION

Dr. Richard Bandler, co-founder of NLP (Neuro-Linguistic Programming, which is a component of many energy techniques) says, *"My job is to chide people into new ways of thinking and new ways of acting so that they can have more fun in life and get more stuff done."*

To piggyback on his words, it isn't my job to chide and guide people to new ways of thinking and new ways of acting so that they can have more fun in life.

It's more than my job. It's my joy and my passion. There is nothing to compare with that love, deep trust and connection that grows out of helping others along their healing journey.

And now, on to why you may not be getting the results you want from tapping and what to do about it to transform your world.

PART I:

23 Reasons Why Transformation Is Such a Challenge

Reason #1:

We Have Subconscious Imprints

The reason we have problems
is that we were born.

Dr. Richard Bandler, Founder, NLP

Early life events over which we had no control and which we had no way to put into perspective at such a young age can become etched into our minds and set the theme for our lives.

I will illustrate what I mean with a rather complicated example from my own history that until recently affected every aspect of my financial life and that still runs interference from time to time.

If you read the testimonials on my websites[i], you will see that my ability to generate ideas for my corporate clients has made hundreds of millions of dollars for them over the years. I have always been successful at producing results—for other people.

This created the illusion of career success. But for myself, life was a pattern of financial pain and hardship, financial gains and losses.

Thirty-five years of one therapy after another—including a three-year stint studying Gestalt Therapy. Over $100,000 spent in search of a solution and still the pattern persisted.

Then, one day, I was casually telling a good friend this story from my childhood:

I was born on the Canadian Prairies where, it is said, you can sit on your porch and watch your dog running away from home. For days. My grandparents were homesteaders who had lived through the depression of the Dirty 30's. Money was scarce. But my father inherited, and then sold, the family farm and we moved to the big city of Edmonton, Alberta. From there, we moved to a god-forsaken little community in Northern Alberta when I was just-turned-five.

My father had invested his farm inheritance in the purchase of a hotel in McLennan, Alberta with a partner. At his instruction, my mother had bought enough clothes and toys for her three children to last two years.

In early July, family and furnishings moved into the hotel.

Imprinted Memories

Within the month, disaster struck. My most vivid childhood memory (and I have precious few) happens in the back seat of my father's brand new Studebaker, in the pre-dawn hours of a hot summer's night, frozen in horror as the flames devour our home, furniture, clothes, cash, family memorabilia and source of income. Although that would not enter a five-year-old's mind. (My personal tragedy was that I had lost a brand new baby doll).

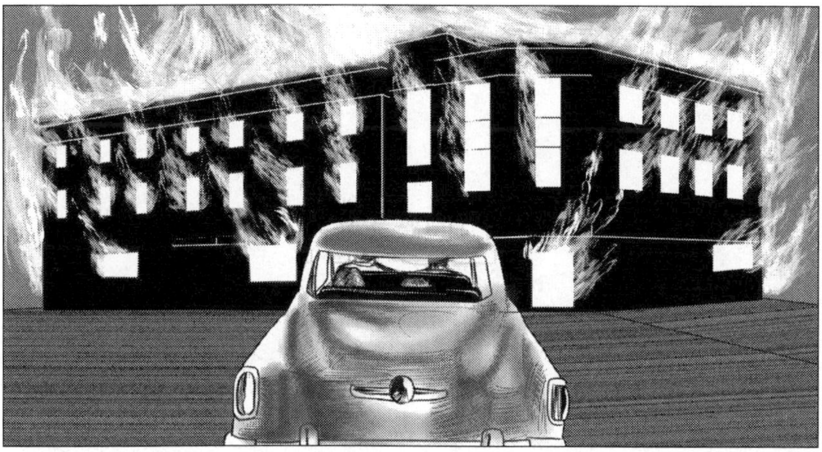

That is my most vivid childhood memory, at age five, sitting on the edge of the back seat of the family car with my older sister, having been rescued from the blaze, wearing only little white summer panties, witnessing our new "home" go up in flames.

My father's coping mechanism was to cuss and swear in taboo church terms. (Anyone of French Canadian heritage will know exactly what I mean!) My mother sobbed uncontrollably. My older sister slept. (This is a story in itself because my sister has been singularly unaffected by events that traumatized my early years.)

My father had rescued me and my sister but by the time he returned for my little brother the room was engulfed in flames. The floor had collapsed. You can imagine my parents' agony until they learned hours later that their little boy had been saved by a nurse who was a guest in the hotel that night.

The fire had started in a coal bin in the basement. To make things worse, there was no water to extinguish the flames because the town's water supply came to this desolate place only every so often, by freight car.

Unquenched, the embers smoldered for a month. Or perhaps that was just a family's distorted memory. Perhaps it was just days or weeks.

To a child it was forever.

I remember walking past the scorching rubble some time later and my three-year-old brother's tears at seeing the remains of his little red wagon in the smoldering ashes.

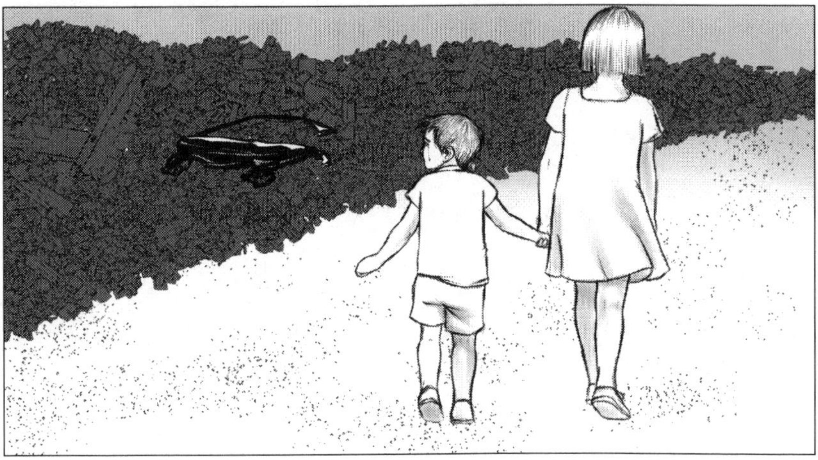

Our family of five lived on charity in a two-room shack with no running water, a pot-bellied stove, and icicles on the inside walls in winter. (Do you know how cold it gets in Northern Alberta? So cold you can get frostbite on your nose on the 2-block walk to school.)

Bricks were scarce because of a building boom and my mother sold reclaimed bricks from the hotel ruins to put food on the table.

There ensued an ugly lawsuit with the insurance company whose position was that the fire had been intentionally set.

Eventually, the suit was settled. Soon after the hotel was rebuilt my family moved to the Great Lakes region of Canada.

WHAT WAS LOST IN THE FIRE? A LOT MORE THAN DOLLS AND LITTLE RED WAGONS.

There I was, telling my story. And then my friend said ...

> *Think of the emotional message you got when you were little: "everything goes up in smoke." That set the theme for your life. You work and work and work. You put your life energy into it and everything you accomplish goes up in smoke. That's your pattern. What was really going on with you was the emotional connection to money – loneliness, destruction, powerlessness and aborted plans.*

Then she listed events from my life. [This girl forgets nothing. So as not to confuse, what you see in parentheses are my responses to her insights.]

> *Your dream of a career as a concert pianist came to an end at age 17 when your father declared bankruptcy. You missed out on a full university scholarship by point-something because you got sick during final grade XIII exams. You turned down the opportunity of a full Ph. D. fellowship to please your husband who didn't want to live with a student for the next few years and said it was time for you to get a job.*
>
> *You worked for nine years in a business with your husband and walked away from the marriage with only $500 in shares for all your efforts. And that business still provides him a millionaire lifestyle?* [Hardly seems fair, does it?]

How many times have your own businesses failed? [Now you're touching too close to the bone!]

Didn't you take on a business partner who – on the very day you succeeded in landing a cross-country training gig with one of Canada's leading financial companies – announced that he was going back to the position he had held before joining forces with you? [How dare he?]

How many times have you won the contract, only to see it go up in smoke for no apparent reason? [Too many. The most recent being the financial collapse of late 2008 that took my Asia consulting business with it.]

How many lawsuits have you been involved in? [OMG!]

How many career changes have you had? [8, 9, 10?]

How many times have you invested in properties only to sell them at a loss? [Four]

How many times has your property been destroyed by an outside source, rodents or broken water pipes? [That would be four as well.]

Everything that happened after that was repetition of a pattern.

So what's my point? Other than the fact that it wasn't easy being me?

Sometimes the imprint is so deep it's out of our grasp.

I'm a trained practitioner, for crying out loud. I had decades of talk therapy. Studied three years to become a Gestalt Therapist.

Became certified in Three-In-One Concepts, studied NLP and immersed myself in various meridian tapping techniques.

And yet, I never saw the connection between my repetitive patterns and something that etched into my mind at the age of five.

All my life's themes were set in place. Boom. Bust. Boom. Business failure. Problems with insurance companies. Accidents. Legal hassles. Delays. Aborted plans. A 9-year bout with Fibromyalgia that I've written about elsewhere and that brought me to my knees financially.[ii] All seemingly outside my control.

But most of all … most of all … you work and work, you build, and suddenly and overnight, you can just lose everything. Then you keep repeating the pattern.

> *Life going up in smoke. Everything in your life goes up in smoke. You set your pattern right there, that's what life is all about. Work hard and lose everything. It will go up in smoke. You will be helpless. You will be powerless.*
>
> *You've decided you're not going to reach the lofty goals, so you unknowingly do things that stop you, that block you, that cause you to miss opportunities or you find opportunities that give you the desired disastrous results.*

Not All Imprints Are Negative

At my father's Celebration of Life ceremony eight years ago, my brother told a story he had never told before. His account shows how happy and repetitive early childhood experiences also etch into our subconscious minds and shape our lives.

He talked about his joy as a young boy of going to the hotel in Niagara Falls with his father every Sunday morning because he was allowed to keep whatever coins he found in the bar.

We had by now relocated to Ontario where my father had invested in another hotel. Things were booming due to the massive Niagara hydroelectric power project. Away from home, the workers celebrated pay day by drinking up on Friday and Saturday nights.

They didn't bother with the loose change, it seems.

My brother laughingly said, *"That's how I became* mercenary. *I developed the belief that money was everywhere! I still believe that money is everywhere*!"

And for him, it is. It's part of his DNA.

Dynamic of Cellular Memory

Our subconscious literally runs 95% of our life. It runs our life through beliefs – positive and negative – that we hold at a cellular level. For many of us, that means our lives are being run by a 5-year old.

I will have more to say on this topic in Reason #21: We got hijacked by the beliefs of a child.

For a deeper discussion of the concept of patterns, see Reason #2: We tend to focus on the symptoms rather than the underlying patterns which are the unseen causes of our discomfort.

Perhaps you also had an early life experience that determined your destiny. Positively or negatively. If so, I would love to hear your story. Who knows, I may write another book!

You can reach me directly: mia@miadoucet.com

Reason #2:

We Tend to Focus on the Symptoms Rather Than the Underlying Patterns Which Are the Unseen Causes of Our Discomfort

Like most Western medicine, when we work on our own schtuff we tend to focus on the symptoms (the seen cause) not the root cause of the problem.

We tend to focus on what we see in our external world rather than focusing on our internal world, where we make things happen.

We're not aware of the invisible process, only the external, visible results.

The Unseen Cause: Unconscious Programming

Our brain keeps recreating pictures and sensations from memories of previous experiences, often from our early childhood when we were too young to take charge of our lives.

The pictures, sensations and deep emotional triggers continue to play in our minds 24-hours-a-day. Non-stop. Round-the-clock. That is the unconscious negative programming that is running our life.

It explains why, after a certain age, we begin to see distinct differences between the patterns in our own life and other people's lives.

Speaking of patterns, did you know that detailed, never-ending patterns exist in all of nature as well as abstract mathematical equations? They are called fractals.

More on fractals in a moment. First, let's look a bit further into unconscious programming.

THE INVISIBLE TUG-OF-WAR

Now here's the thing. You and I have both a conscious mind and an unconscious mind. (I also believe we have a super-conscious mind that connects us to a higher, collective consciousness that we call God or Creator or Source or The Universe or any of a myriad of names.) But that's a conversation for another time.

If our conscious mind wants one thing (I just want a loving relationship) and our subconscious mind wants another (I confuse love with neglect because that's how I was treated as a small child), we're going to have conflict. That inner conflict will show up in our life as self-sabotage or resistance or powerlessness or addiction to the dark side of love.

At the very least, it's going to show up as not getting what we say we want. Or getting what we say we don't want.

THE MIGHTY UNCONSCIOUS

Decades ago, brain scientists at Yale and Stanford determined that our mind is like an iceberg. We are unaware of 95% of what drives us because that 95% is submerged and below our conscious awareness.

Because the subconscious is so much more powerful than the conscious, when there is conflict the subconscious wins every time.

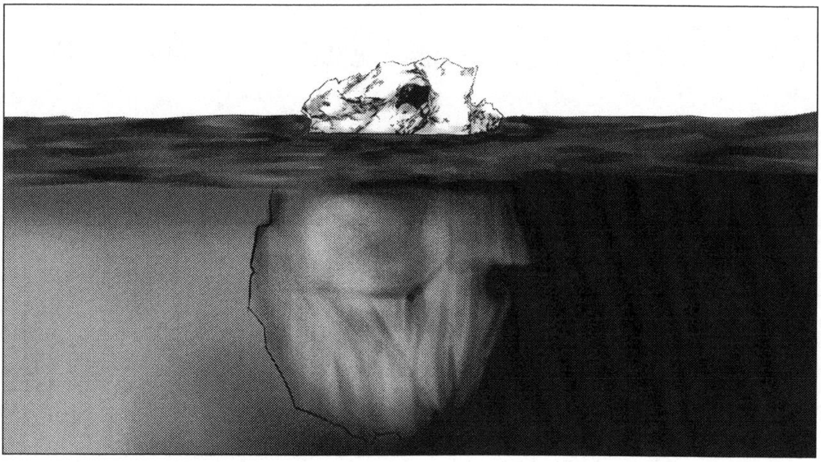

In contrast to the power of the conscious mind, the subconscious mind is a million times more powerful an information processor. Also, as neuroscientists emphasize, the conscious mind provides 5% or less of the cognitive activity during the day. Ninety-five to ninety-nine percent of our behavior is directly derived from the subconscious.

BRUCE H. LIPTON, PH.D., AUTHOR, THE BIOLOGY OF BELIEF

THE ROOT CAUSE – PERPETUAL PATTERNS

Fractals are repetitions of simple patterns. Said another way, fractals are simple patterns that repeat themselves. I think of them as echoes. A simple pattern that echoes or repeats itself often enough creates an infinitely complex pattern.

> *A fractal is a never-ending pattern. Fractals are infinitely complex patterns that are self-similar across different scales. They are created by repeating a simple process over and over in an ongoing feedback loop.*[iii]

FRACTALS IN NATURE

Spheres, spiral patterns (galaxies, hurricanes, seashells), splashes (think of pebbles dropped into a pond), waves, snowflakes, crystals, clouds, mountain ranges, branching patterns (rivers and streams, trees, plants and algae). Veins in plant leaves and in our lungs, feet and hands. Even the genome has a highly organized structure.

You get the idea, fractal patterns are everywhere in nature.

FRACTALS IN MATHEMATICS

Fractals are the basis of computer-based modelling. "Abstract fractals can be generated by a computer calculating a simple equation over and over."[iv]

And how does this relate to the subject at hand?

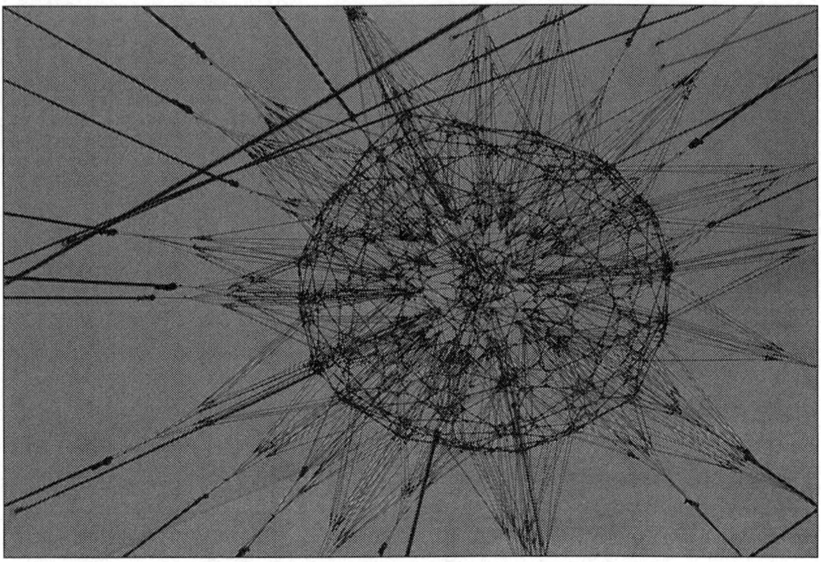

THIS INTRIGUINGLY TITLED PHOTO "GALAXIES ... OR A VIRUS?" IS BY MARARIE[v]

You have often read that our mind is like a computer. (Of course, it's more accurate to say that the computer is like the human mind, because the mind came first. But you know what I mean.)

In childhood, we soak in our culture and environment. We absorb the language, world views, mental attitudes and ways of thinking. They become the mind's software.

My theory is that the patterns we acquire in childhood set the core, imprinted beliefs that fix the context of our life (issues such as deservingness, attitudes toward money, and self-worth to mention just a few).

Like a computer calculating a simple equation without stop, we keep recreating our patterns in an endless feedback loop until we take charge of our subconscious mind to interrupt the cycle and create new patterns.

When you think you got rid of a problem and it reappears in a problem somewhere else. When you are unable to rid yourself of certain patterns in your life, no matter what you try. When you have not had success with meridian tapping methods, you may well be right to blame it on fractals.

HERE'S WHAT YOU NEED TO KNOW ...

The subconscious makes sure our fractals are self-repairing. Since the subconscious always has a good positive reason for any of our patterns, it will do whatever it needs to in order to perpetuate and reconstruct a fractal. Unless the loop is completely broken we will continue to revert to the old negative programming.

GET THE MOST OUT OF YOUR TAPPING EFFORTS

We need to get to the root of the problem which is often hidden and lost in the past. The only remedy I can see is to break and delete the negative fractal.

In Part III, I outline my own, unscientific, untested experiment for doing this on your own. I would be very interested to hear if and how it works for you.

Reason #3:

We're Unable to Get to the Structure of the Problem on Our Own

When a client presents a problem (broken relationships/unresolved anger/whatever the issue), my first task as a practitioner is to figure out what the person is doing inside their head/mind/body to create and construct a situation that presents itself as the problem.

My second task is to disrupt the brain's repetitive patterns that keep the problem alive. That's where tapping comes in. For tapping to work you have to step inside the mind.

It is rather difficult for us to step into our own mind and start operating within our way of processing thoughts in order to change bad memories. Most of us don't get that it is our internal processing that creates problems in our life.

If we subscribe to the concept that the past is past and only the present moment is real, then how does the mind keep re-creating the problem? We must be doing something internally to keep a problem alive.

How did the subconscious mind encode the event? How does it continue to keep it alive?

If we can figure *that* out, if we can get to the structure of it, we can dismantle the problem for good.

Working on myself and others, it has been most useful to treat each memory as a figment of the mind. This takes a certain amount of detachment.

Working on your own, it's very helpful to think in terms of what we are doing inside our head to make our problem feel real in the moment.

Let's say your "problem" is depression or anxiety. Your response to the following questions will reveal the mental structure that is creating your world: *"How do you know? What tells you you're depressed or anxious? Do you see a picture in your mind? Do you hear sounds inside your head? Is it a feeling in your body?"*

The practitioner can see how you are successfully producing your depression or anxiety or whatever the problem may be. (To you it appears to be a problem that is out of your control but we say that in fact your mind is successfully producing and reproducing a certain result.) So it is in your control. That's wonderful news, actually. If it's in my control, I can do something about it.

You don't just want to do away with a negative feeling. You want to keep it from recurring.

So what am I doing to *produce* depression? What am I doing to produce anxiety? What am I doing to keep this anger at my mother alive?

To find that out, it's useful to . . .

STEP INTO YOUR MEMORY

Some people think that memories are like movies that play inside your head. That in order to remember an event you have to see it in your mind's eye. I used to think that and it was very frustrating because at that time I had no visual memory at all.

But that impression was false. A feeling is a memory. Thoughts, spoken and unspoken words, sounds, smells, tastes and sensations are memories. They are held in the body at a cellular level. That is why replaying the memory causes a physical response or symptom(s) in the body. When we focus the tapping on those physical responses (as opposed to scripted language) we start to disrupt the brain's repetitive patterns that keep problems alive.

CHILDHOOD MEMORIES HOLD THE CLUE

What is important to understand when wanting to get to the structure of the problem is HOW we as a child represented and responded to an event in our mind and body. The decisions we made at an early age, when we had no context, no frame of reference, no life experience from which to put things into perspective; when we didn't have the language to express what we felt.

I do not suggest that you work alone on traumatic and deeply upsetting life episodes because it is not so easy to detach ourselves. There is a danger of causing a painful overreaction. In these instances, you will want to work with a skilled practitioner.

For less intrusive memories, you may find useful the 9-Step process to clear the structure of a problem (Part III).

Reason #4:

We Get Overwhelmed

I feel like I'm unraveling on the inside.

James (a client)

Free content on the Internet is wonderful. And no one gives more excellent free content than media-savvy practitioners. The resources are endless. But …

What most of us need is an objective, trained guide to provide clarity and help us identify the underlying patterns that cause us to repeat the same undesired results in our lives.

This was the topic of Reason #2: We tend to focus on the symptoms rather than the underlying patterns which are the unseen causes of our discomfort.

What's in Your Emotional Ocean?

Some of us live our days and nights with a low-level dread. We work to suppress emotions as a way of coping. Working on our own emotions can open us to feelings of anxiety and panic.

One of the reasons it's painful to work with our own emotions is that once we skim off the superficial stuff and suppressed memories and feelings start coming to the surface, we can find ourselves lost. When we don't know what to do with those feelings, it can be overwhelming.

First of all, there are some emotions we would just rather not have or acknowledge. Some are just too fearful, too painful or too intimidating to delve into on our own.

It's hard to dive into our own emotional ocean without fearing we might drown.

It is my job, and that of any practitioner, to reduce the level of fear and resistance, throughout the entire clearing process.

After we worked together, a client wrote to me that she had "*tried everything I could think of to overcome my health issues, which included my emotional state. I was feeling anxious, overwhelmed, depleted, trapped, imploded and I wanted to get back to feeling energized and confident. I was really in a negative zone and didn't know how to break free of it. I had been reading everything I could get my hands on regarding The Law of Attraction. Nothing was working. I could tap for an hour and not feel a release.*"

Clearing her overwhelm was a six-month project.

If, like this person, you have had a nervous breakdown. If you are feeling anxious, overwhelmed, depleted, trapped and imploded and want to free your life of negativity, you too will most likely require the help of a skilled practitioner.

However, if you feel you can do the work on your own and are committed to doing so, here's a suggestion to reduce the overwhelm …

Isolate each negative emotion and connect it to specific memories. Focus on *one* emotion and *one* memory at a time. Don't try to "boil the ocean" as one of my clients would say. [See Part III: Give context to negative emotions.]

Reason #5:

Our Brain Went into Shock to Help Us Cope

When something traumatic happens to us, the basic instinct to survive kicks in to protect us mentally, physically or both.

If you think about it, if we don't cope and survive the short term, the long term is irrelevant.

But today's solution will be tomorrow's problem.

Body Shock

While my son was completing his Ph.D. thesis at the University of Amsterdam, he and a team of colleagues went to Praia das Maçãs, Portugal for a technical conference. Off hours, they took to the beach.

Andrés swam out too far and got sucked down and out to sea by an undertow. Friends and strangers attempted repeatedly to rescue him, without success.

In the meantime, his friend Stephanie was told by a nearby fisherman that the only way to get back safely was to swim toward the rockbound part of the coast.

With a surge of adrenaline, Andrés managed to extricate himself and swim to safety, encouraged and guided by Stephanie's frantic jumping jacks on the shore.

His legs collapsed as he touched bottom. His friends carried him onto the beach and he was taken to hospital by ambulance. After disgorging "a load of sea water" Andrés felt better and managed to persuade the doctor to let him return to the hotel.

The next morning he was again rushed to hospital by ambulance. His internal organs had shut down.

Survival mode had kicked in.

Doctors told him that all his reserves of energy had gone to his leg and arm muscles in order to make available every ounce of strength to meet the urgent need to save his life. He handled the immediate trauma extremely well. But in the process his internal organs had been depleted of their energy supply. After a two-week hospital stay he was back to normal.

So with physical trauma, the organs shut down in order to keep us alive. A parallel phenomenon happens when our subconscious perceives we can't handle an emotional trauma. The brain will go into survival mode in order to protect our cognitive and neurological coping mechanisms from overwhelm.

BRAIN SHOCK THEORY

When the brain experiences a shock from out of left field it compartmentalizes all component aspects of the incident. Sights are stored in one place. Sounds in another. Smells, physical sensations, thoughts and feelings as well. The brain splits them off to different areas so we won't be overwhelmed and unable to handle the impact of the trauma.

After the immediate danger goes away the information stays compartmentalized and doesn't naturally get integrated. The brain gets stuck, in a sense.

Then when something similar to the original incident happens the brain reacts the same way. It places the component aspects into these same compartments. Again, the experience doesn't get processed.

We disassociate.

This is the opposite of what happens when "neurons that fire together wire together." [Discussed in Reason #7: It's etched on our mental hard drive.] Because in the instance of brain shock, we're not in fact reliving the episode. We have *forgotten* the episode. If remembered, we may refer to it in an offhand way.

While it doesn't overwhelm us it still has an impact on our life from the point of view that we can't move beyond it. We may get triggered by a sight or sound or sensation but we are unable to connect the dots to make sense of it.

The problem is, when we're trying to work through a situation on our own, we either don't remember the significant event or we think about it in such a nonchalant way that its importance never enters our mind.

We never get to tap on the deep emotion, which is essential to tapping success.

It takes an objective person who is skilled at hearing what is not being said to put the parts together again.

In retrospect, brain shock would explain what happened in my five-year-old brain when I witnessed a blazing fire under highly charged circumstances.

It would explain the impact on my entire life. It would also explain my detached, dissociated attitude in recalling the memory.

Until a few years ago I felt the only impact the fire had on my life was that I had to start school one year ahead of schedule, with the result that I never caught up to my classmates physically and emotionally and always felt behind socially and academically.

In writing this section, I realize that, to this day, I cannot summon any emotion about the fire. Which of course means I will need the services of a good practitioner.

Reason #6:

We May Be in a State of Trance and Not Realize It

I AM ALWAYS AT A LOSS TO KNOW
HOW MUCH TO BELIEVE OF MY OWN STORIES.

Washington Irving, American author, essayist, biographer, historian, and diplomat (1783 –1859)

LET ME BEGIN by saying that trance is an activity you and I do naturally.

We're not referring to a state that is induced by a hypnotist swinging a pendulum on a chain. We're not referring to anything as dramatic as being mesmerized by a blazing fire. We're talking about a state that we easily slip into, many times a day, most often without noticing.

A trance is something we do automatically without thought or effort because we're just so good at it. Our brains get really, really good at anything we constantly practice or rehearse.

PROBLEMS ARE HYPNOTIC STATES

When we step into a familiar memory we slip into a well-rehearsed, trance-like state.

A word, a facial expression, a scent, a flowering tree, anything can pull us back into an earlier time with all its associated emotions.

Incidentally, TV advertisements are designed to put us into a state of trance. That's how they get us to buy things we don't need and crave foods that aren't good for us, distort our bodies and give us grief.

Think of a trance as anything going through our mind that is not happening to us right here, right now, in the flesh, in the present moment.

By that definition, most of us are in a state of trance most of the time. (How many people do you know who live life in the present moment? *Do you know any*?)

THE LIGHTS ARE ON BUT NOBODY'S HOME

Every time we replay a memory or a conversation—positive or negative, real or imaginary; every time we focus on a problem or start to envision or worry about the future; every time we are not consciously present in the moment, we are in a state of trance. Our body is present but our thoughts are elsewhere.

It's so easy to go into a trance. And if we don't even know we're in trance, it's pretty darn difficult to pull ourselves out.

Even if we know what's going on it's hard for us to enter into our own trance in order to change and rewrite a memory.

Good and Bad Trances

There are good trances and bad trances and the good trances are no problem at all. The bad trances are the cause of our unhappiness.

What qualifies as a bad trance? I would say a bad trance is any thought that robs us of being happy in the present moment.

- a negative emotional sequence
- a negative movie that plays over and over in our head
- a never-ending, imaginary conversation or argument that runs through our mind without resolution
- a negative physical sensation that happens whenever we replay an unhappy memory

It isn't the actual negative events that we experienced that cause havoc. It's the fact that we didn't shrug them off, the way geese do when they go their own way honking and hissing after a squabble.

It's the *replaying* of negative experiences that causes havoc.

If you're still furious about something that happened 19 years ago you can bet you're in the deep, deep groove of a negative trance.

To Us the Memories Are Real

I'm reminded of a recent client, "Sandra," who herself was a trained therapist and who had never succeeded in overcoming a faint and distant memory of early childhood sexual abuse, either working on her own or with several other therapists.

We had no sooner started our first session than Sandra fell into a deep trance of herself at a very young age.

Deep in her trance she sobbed, trembled uncontrollably and visibly regressed to a terrified four-year-old.

As I watched, the thought grew that this emotional state of terror was very, very familiar to her. At the risk of sounding mean, I suspected that this state had been very well rehearsed over years of talk therapy.

Clearly, she was reliving in the present tense an event or series of events from her early childhood as though those events were real in the present tense, which they were not. In present time she was perfectly safe in my office. All grown up and a successful professional in her early 40's.

There is no way that she could have ever worked her way out of the familiar groove on her own—despite an advanced degree in psychotherapy.

Compassion Hazard

Even practitioners can slip into your trance and have *too much empathy.* I imagine this is one reason Sandra's previous therapies had not created positive change.

I recently heard a veteran EFT practitioner say this in a radio interview:

"It's difficult for the facilitator to sit in the discomfort. We want to get out of it as soon as possible." And, *"It's our own discomfort over their discomfort that causes us to rush into offering positives."*

If the person you are working with has your issues and identifies with you, empathizes with you or is unable to guide you through the rough spots, your issues will not go away because that person now becomes part of the problem.

If a facilitator rushes into offering positives before a matter has been resolved because of our own discomfort, it means we have bought into your story and slipped into your trance.

If I am in the trance with a client, or if I am uncomfortable with his discomfort, I'm going to be there too soon with reassuring words, positive reframes or matrix reimprinting.

But a good practitioner treats the hurtful memory as a *fabrication*, not real. The idea is that it's all illusion, because it is not happening in the present. It does not exist. The only way something that happened in the past can exist in the present is for you and me to keep recreating it.

That's one of the benefits of working with a good practitioner. We don't buy into the client's trance. We can only help you when we stand outside your story and lead you safely out of your hypnotic trance state. That's our job.

Taking Trance to the Extreme

There once was a video on YouTube (I would direct you to it but sadly, it is no longer available) in which Dr. Richard Bandler, co-founder of Neuro-linguistic programming, tells the priceless story of treating an institutionalized man who insisted he was the one true Jesus Christ.

As best I can remember, and missing some of the details, it went something along these lines ...

Bandler: *Are you Jesus?*

Man: *Yes, my son.*

Bandler: *I'll be back in a minute.*

Bandler returns with a measuring tape. He asks the man to hold out his arms, and proceeds to measure the length of his arms and his height from toe to top of head. Then he leaves.

He returns a while later with a hammer, some long, sharp nails, and some boards. He starts to pound them into the form of a cross. To heighten the tension, he calls in some hired actors dressed as roman centurions.

Man: *What are you doing?*

Bandler: *Are you Jesus?*

Man: *Yes, my son.*

Bandler: [Continuing to pound a nail] *Then you know why I'm here.*

Man [wondrously popping out of his trance]: *I'm not Jesus Christ! I'm not Jesus Christ!*

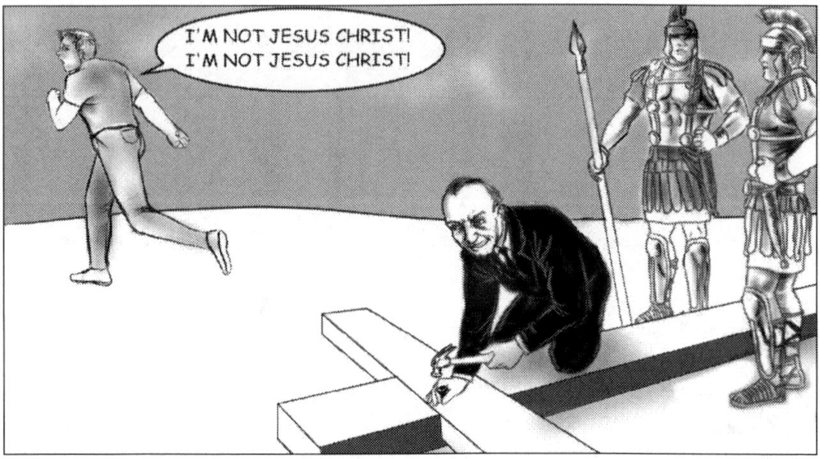

Hopefully this recounting doesn't offend your sensibilities. It's such a splendid illustration of the power of trance and the power of the practitioner standing outside the story yet entering the client's world. Operating within the belief system that created it. Dealing with the story as not real – a hypnotic trance state – and using the person's subconscious belief system to bring about a dramatic cure.

Such brilliance.

Reason #7:

It's Etched on Our Mental Hard Drive

Neurons that fire together
wire together

This catchy little phrase by Canadian neuro-psychologist Donald Hebb dates back to 1949.

Hebb found that when neurons fire in sequence they fuse together in such a way that actions and thinking patterns become habitual. Every time we repeat a motion or thought or action or feeling, we strengthen the connection between the neurons (brain cells).

Muscle Memory

This is wonderful when we're learning to play tennis and practice ensures that muscle memory will kick in when we need all brain and body parts to fire off in the right sequence at the time the ball is in position to be hit.

Not so wonderful when we're trying to build new habits and the old grooves of the neural pathways keep us stuck because muscle memory guarantees that when we relive a past event in memory, or worry about something that might happen in the future the same neurons will fire off, in the same sequence, with the same emotional results.

We Play Our Patterns

We're successfully producing problems in the present because we keep rehearsing our narrative of events from the past. We've recreated it so often in our minds that we've kept the neurons firing. We've kept it alive.

I suppose the wiring together is what causes OCD (Obsessive Compulsive Disorder). One man said to me, "I can't stop the record. It's always there. I'm driving my car and it's there. I wake up in the morning and it's there."

So if you want to break a deeply etched pattern such as an out-of-control craving, it's a good idea to get the neurons sparking in sequence before you start tapping.

Here's an example of what I mean.

I had a client – "Margaret" – who wanted to overcome her addiction to sugar mixed with peanut butter, as well as Hershey's chocolate. For years she had tried unsuccessfully on her own to kick the habit.

In a group session, I asked her to show me what she did as she was preparing to enjoy her sugar-encrusted peanut butter treat every night. She curled up on the sofa and placed a pillow between her knees the way she always did to watch television. Then she scooped peanut butter from the jar with a spoon and sprinkled sugar on top.

Me: *"Think of how good this is going to make you feel. Smell it. Taste it. Yum. Yum. Yum."*

She easily slips into her trance and we start tapping. [If you missed the conversation about trance, you will find it in Reason #6: We may be in a state of trance and not realize it.]

There's an interesting little sequel to this tale. We didn't get to work on the chocolate because by the time we were done with the first two menaces, she couldn't stand the thought of continuing the process with another beloved treat. And I caved in to her whim, thinking it would be too cruel to continue.

Margaret tells me that, to this day, she still can't stand even the sight of a peanut butter jar. But she is still hooked on Hershey's chocolate and will have to come to my next group session to rid herself of the craving.

We're So Funny!

Telling you Margaret's story reminds me of a woman I worked with years ago who wanted to lose 30 pounds. One of the things "Grace" was addicted to was "Sweet & Salty" bars. She had to have one every day of the week at 10 o'clock in the morning, whether at work or on weekends. We took care of that in one session.

The next week I asked how she was doing with the "Sweet & Salty" craving. She looked at me as though I was out of my mind and with a flick of the wrist and rolling of the eyes, she said:

> *Why are we even having this conversation? They could be in the cupboard until the cows come home. I have no problem with Sweet & Salty bars. They mean nothing to me!*

But in the meantime Grace had developed a lust for anything pure sugar. We took care of that in a second session.

The following week, we had to work on all things salty, like potato chips. We took care of that.

Then didn't she develop a hankering for greasy foods.

Gary Craig talks about "Chasing the Pain." This was more like Chasing the Memory in the Muscles.

How to Cure a Craving on Your Own ...

For best results, make sure you address – in specific – each and every delicious subversive thing about the substance you want out of your life. For example, if you are hooked on donuts, call up every aspect of the donut that calls out to you: the look of it, the aroma, the anticipation, the flavor, the texture as you bite into it.

Otherwise, your subconscious mind will find a way to help you feed your craving (which is not really about food anyway).

Then catch yourself if, like Grace, other food itches develop. Work on every aspect of the new craving.

You May Experience Resistance

And don't be afraid to test later by tempting yourself with the food. Testing won't compromise the results. If the craving is still there, keep at it until you feel totally free of it.

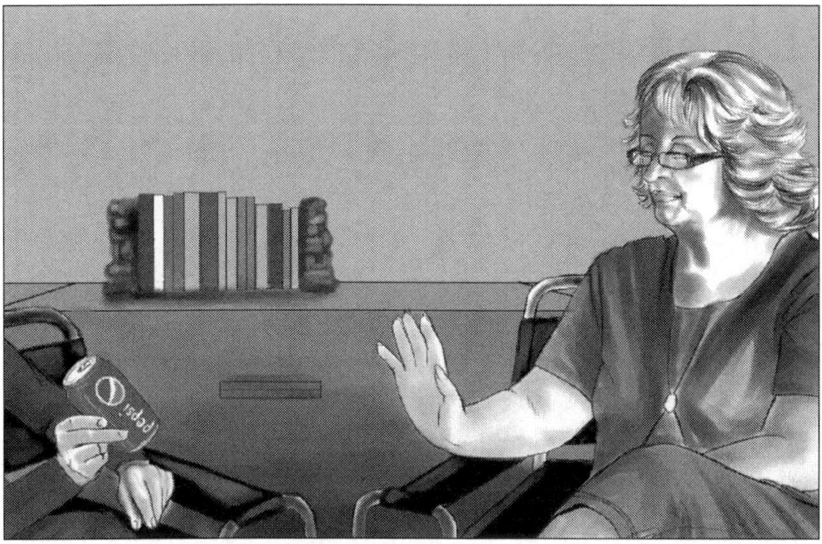

If you like videos, there's an entertaining little 7:49-minute YouTube video in which I help my client work through her sadness over giving up her "old friend" Diet Pepsi.[vi] [To access the video: Type Mia Doucet Goodbye To An Addiction in the search bar. You will love her reaction at the 5-minute mark.]

Reason #8:

Our Uniqueness

The problem with the galaxy of information available today on meridian tapping is that none of it is personalized and customized to **you**. How could it be when you're not the person receiving the treatment?

While I agree that we can gain a lot of understanding – not to mention compassion – by viewing other people's sessions. And while a lot of practitioners believe in the EFT concept of "Borrowed Benefits" and no one can dispute that some people do benefit vicariously some of the time. And while we are not alone with respect to problems we may have, each of us has our own unique context, our own life experiences, our own memories, and our own internal references to deal with.

Our experiences are encoded in our mind in our own unique way. We are unique in the way we process, record and store information, retrieve memories, interpret past events and hold on to past hurts. And we develop different ways of coping with those experiences.

We also have our own way of representing those memories and experiences as physical sensations in our body.

We have different mental constructs that shape our world view. By mental constructs I mean the things we build our life on. We all perceive things differently.

Each family may have its own set of "rules." (Even so, if you have brothers and sisters, do you sometimes find it hard to believe that they were born to the same parents? I do.)

Are those videos personalized to you? Do they help you get to the heart of your own life drama? Do they teach you how to clear out the core beliefs that keep you repeating the same patterns, ad nauseum?

Usually not.

"EFT IN A BOX"

Gary Craig, founder of EFT (Emotional Freedom Techniques) sees a real problem with the generic tapping scripts that many EFT practitioners use in YouTube videos, seminars, webinars, summits and symposiums. He feels that these "global" approaches work for a small minority of people but not for the great majority as they are too generalized to uncover the unconscious programming that is running our lives.

I couldn't agree more.

> *The allure to these scripts involves a convenience factor wherein a ready-made approach is provided that requires no customization or detective work. Just tap on the EFT points while repeating words that someone else provides. Easy. It's a one-size-fits-all or "EFT in a Box" approach.*
>
> GARY CRAIG, FOUNDER, OPTIMAL EFT™

"LOST IN MY OWN LITTLE WORLD... "

I worked with a woman, "Jennifer," who has invested in group teleseminars, webinars and in-person events with practitioners whose names you would recognize in a heartbeat.

She had been tapping along for over a year but was, in her words, *"Lost in my own little world of tapping. I can't seem to get results from it. I believe in it but I don't see the results in it."*

Jennifer had been tapping on the relationship with her mother, what she described as a "severe drinking problem," and her loneliness without a man in her life.

"I give myself permission to release all loneliness." And *"Even though I'm really lonely, I love and accept myself."* And all the other lovely phrases she was saying were not cutting it.

We worked through three significant life episodes from her past involving her mother. In each case, Jennifer's level of emotional intensity went from 10 (very high) to zero.

But it was not until we tapped on, *"I let go all fear that I will always be lonely"* that the tears began to pour.

That was the issue. It was *unique* to her. Not just, I am really lonely. But I am really lonely *and my deepest fear is that I will* always *be lonely.*

GET THE MOST OUT OF YOUR TAPPING EFFORTS

As Gary Craig says, the key here is "to uncover the unconscious programming that is running (our life)."

Precisely because the programming is unconscious, it can be extremely difficult to do on our own.

However, if you're wanting to do it on your own, do what Gary calls …

THE DETECTIVE WORK:

1. Ask yourself:

   What am I really angry about?
   What am I hiding from myself?
   What would I rather not see?

2. Don't concern yourself with words or scripts.

3. Just tap on the sensation itself.

REASON #9:

THE UNCONSCIOUS MIND IS RESISTANT AND PROTECTIVE

ONE OF THE things that is so fascinating about this work is the major role that resistance plays when we attempt to make even minor changes in our lives that we perceive as positive.

As we get close to a resolution of any kind, we tend to want to skip over that chunk and move on. Our attention jumps to another memory or another emotion. Or we hit a wall. Or we kid ourselves into thinking the matter has been dealt with.

As we take off a layer we will often work even harder to protect ourselves because, having cleared one thing, something even scarier may surface.

When I'm working with someone, I'm conscious of working through layers of resistance. Behind the resistance is always fear. Pervasive fear.

FEAR KEEPS US SAFE

By now you know that the role of the unconscious mind is to protect us and keep us safe. The process of change threatens our comfort zone. Numerous studies have shown that we are hard-wired to keep ourselves safe. It is our most basic instinct. Understood in that context, resistance is a natural survival mechanism.

Even if our present situation is uncomfortable, it's the devil we know. And the status quo provides us a sense of security. We want that feeling of security at all costs.

So fear is a way of keeping us safe. What a lovely reframe. *Fear is a form of self love.*

UNCONSCIOUS PROTECTION

If there is a natural resistance to getting to the heart of the matter it's no wonder people quit when they are working on their own.

People who don't feel safe in the world may have problems doing this work unassisted.

I worked with a client, "Gail", who had tapped on her own daily for over a year before contacting me. For many months we worked on the underlying causes of her nervous breakdown several years earlier, her depression, Fibromyalgia, anger, and feelings of loss resulting from numerous family betrayals.

Over several sessions, we made headway, but the real breakthrough came only after we finally got to the heart of the matter: a childhood molestation that had been swept under the proverbial carpet because, in her family, "we don't talk about those things."

Once she had let go of the layers of shame and humiliation, we got to the guilt. Now, how could a person possibly feel guilty about something that happened to her before the age of reason, and that she was powerless to prevent?

Well, as Dr. Phil has so often said, "Children have a way of figuring out it's all their fault."

Under the guilt, we uncovered she held a visceral fear of eternal damnation.

Due to Gail's strict, early religious upbringing and beliefs, her subconscious mind was protecting her from the fear of burning in hell for eternity for the abuse she had suffered as a child.

How could a person possibly get to this depth on her own without the guidance of a trusted, objective, non-threatening third party?

WE ARE BLIND TO OUR BLIND SPOTS

Like 100% of the population, we can't see our own blind spots. We may be totally oblivious to them. If we do notice, we may immediately discount what is glaringly obvious to those around us. Because much of what goes on with us is deeply engrained. It's so much a part of our self-concept. And self-concept is not so easy to change.

That's because our deepest beliefs are formed before the age of reason. We come up with conclusions no one suspects could cause problems later in life. These beliefs become the filters through which we view and build our lives.

For more on this topic, see Reason #21: We got hijacked by the beliefs of a child.

THE MANY FACES OF RESISTANCE

This natural resistance makes it much more difficult to work on our own. And it can show up in many forms:

- Feeling overwhelmed at how much there is to tap on.
- Distractions. On our own, it's too easy for us to let ourselves be distracted by related emotions or memories.
- Fear. It might not feel safe to work alone or to work on deeply buried issues, so we quit when we get scared or the pain feels too real.
- Discomfort. When our comfort zone is threatened it raises barriers. We fail to focus our attention on the body's physical response through wanting to avoid discomfort.
- Unwillingness to let go of an emotion such as anger, grief or resentment.
- Unwillingness to forgive.
- Lack of commitment to the process. A part of us desperately wants our life to change. Another part is not so sure.
- Not allowing ourselves to go deep enough. As we remove a chunk or layer we will often work even harder to protect our core.
- Overload. A man recently told me he was unable to do the work on his own because the tapping only surfaced the anger he felt towards members of his family. He was not

able to resolve the anger and that was making life even more difficult.

- A feeling of helplessness. One of my clients said, *"There's a gaping void between knowing what I have to do and being able to do it for myself."*

- Fear of pain. We may be afraid of approaching a matter head on for fear it might hurt. Because we think it might be too painful we fail to allow the feeling to intensify before beginning tapping.

But any discomfort is minimal and lasts only a few moments.

Working through the clearing process is nothing worse than what you put yourself through in your own head day after day. Think of it this way: with these methods, you might just have to go through it again one last time, and then it will be over.

Get the Most out of Your Tapping Efforts

When things aren't budging, you are probably experiencing resistance. Since we give power to whatever we resist it's important to acknowledge and defuse the resistance in order to melt it away.

There are two vastly different approaches to resolving resistance.

One approach is based on Gestalt Therapy's Paradox of Change, which says that we can change only once we fully accept ourselves as we are now.

Just accept yourself.

It's a lovely concept in principal, but one that is not so easy for most of us to do. (It never worked for me.)

If you can't move through the resistance, the alternative is to directly address it head on:

Ask yourself: *Why? Why can't I let this go? What do I get out of it? I must be getting something out of it.*

If that brings up any hesitation or discomfort, ask another question: *What is it about this that it doesn't feel safe?*

I go into this approach in more detail in Part III: Questions to ask yourself if you get stuck, and Part III: When you don't know what to say while tapping.

My best suggestion is to use Ask & Receive:

> *"There is a part of my being that already knows it is safe to allow myself to let this problem go. That part of my being is willing to inform the rest of me now. It is doing so now with grace and ease. My mind, body and spirit are receiving this information now. Information transfer is now complete."*

For a more in-depth explanation of the process, see Part III: Ask & Receive.

Reason #10:

It Can Be Painful to Work with Our Darker Memories and Emotions

THE NIGHTMARE WE FEAR MOST
IS THE ONE WE'VE ALREADY BEEN THROUGH.

Donald Woods Winnicott,
English paediatrician and psychoanalyst

As we touched on in the previous chapter, some people find it difficult to allow themselves to go deeper and get to the root of the emotional discomfort.

It's too painful so let's avoid it.

Deflection can be subtle. As a practitioner, I sometimes look back and realize the client has slipped one by me.

Occasionally I work with a person who is really good at suppressing his or her feelings. Some people numb themselves or disassociate from their feelings (okay, so I have to admit I was one of them!) instead of dealing with deeper emotions. And that can play a large part in conditions such as Fibromyalgia, alcoholism, food and other addictions.

I had to deal with repressed anger, fear, shame and all sorts of other emotions including never having felt wanted or loved as a child.

As you probably know, whatever the strongest emotion is, that's what we will attract to ourselves. If we're not happy with the way our lives are going, and we want positive change, then we have to find a way to deal with it even though to do so may seem too painful at the start.

The Roots of Our Pain

I once worked with a woman, "Chris," who happens to be a competent therapist, on the topic of her addiction to all things sweet and sugary. She described her craving as "desperate longing."

Me: *So what is that desperate longing all about?*

She: *The only thing I can do is put that sweet food inside my mouth.*

Me: *It isn't about icing-sugar-frosted donuts, is it?*

When we started to tap, she was overcome with panic as she recalled her "smothering thing." As she described it, her "crazy mother" [her expression] had attempted to smother her with a pillow while she was an infant in her crib.

It took some time, but we cleared the smothering memory to zero.

Chris contacted me a few days later and said …

> *That was a very clear memory. I've worked on my mother stuff endlessly. You do need to go to someone else to work*

these deep things through. I could never face that alone. I couldn't get to that depth. There you were at the end, saying things, tapping away, being irreverent!

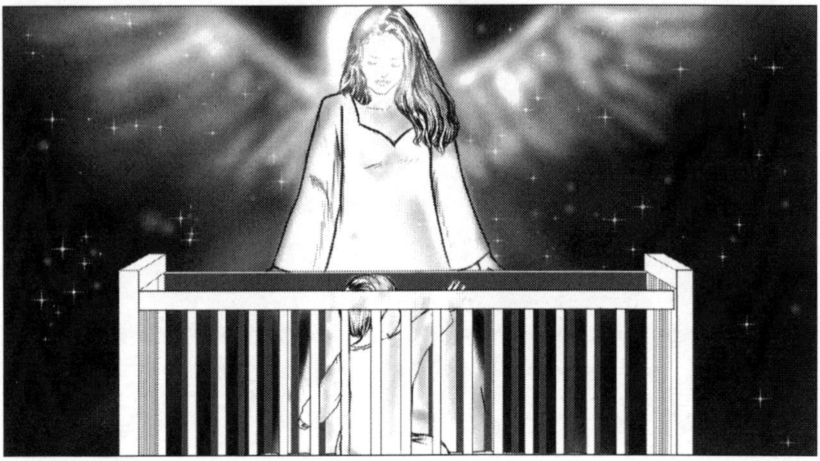

It's only terror.
Let it go.
It's only horror.
Let it go.
It's over.
It's only a memory now.
It doesn't exist anymore.
Time to grow up.
I'm not a baby in a crib.
I'm safe.
I'm all grown up and I'm safe now.
Let it go.

Then you had me re-imprint the memory to what I wish would have happened. I saw an angel standing behind my mother. My mom turned into my angel mom. At the end of it all, I reached out my hand and said, "Oh, mommie!"

And, as often happens, what followed were gales of *"Oh, mommie!"* laughter. No more tears. No more desperate longing. No more addiction to all things sweet and sugary needed to fill a now non-existent emptiness.

Several days later Chris called again and said, *"There is a definite difference. My usual time to eat is 10:00 - 10:30 at night. I actually physically get hungry. You've taken away my craving. I can't even describe how uninterested I am now in eating anything at night. To think, I have worked endlessly on my weight issue."*

GET THE MOST OUT OF YOUR TAPPING EFFORTS

Early stories live in our central nervous system. Your best investment in yourself is to identify, tap on, and clear early childhood events. For most of us, that's where the pain originates.

Reason #11:

We Are Not Connected to the Emotions While Tapping

When triggered, our undesired emotions easily bob up to the surface. But for some of us, when it comes time to work on them, the tendency is to repress, avoid, deny or ignore them.

In fact, undesired emotions may appear to diminish in importance the moment we need to increase their intensity in order to effectively collapse them.

It's just resistance.

The problem is that if we can't access the deep-seated emotions, tapping can't work because what resolves the problem is sparking, focusing and tapping on the raw emotions and the visual, auditory, and physical sensations that associate to the negative memories.

"Joan" had been tapping on her own for two years. Still, a life theme of loneliness and loss persisted. In her words, "*things and people that you love, leave you.*"

Joan's story (as reported by her in an exercise clients do before their first appointment) had provided me a context for her loneliness, feelings of loss and eating to console herself.

Thanks to her permission to let me pique and perturb her a bit, we were able to break through to the repressed emotion.

SOME PEOPLE MAY FIND THIS APPROACH ABRASIVE:

Me: *Go into feeling really lonely and feeling really sorry for yourself.*

She: *I can't.*

Me: *Sure you can. You do it all the time.*

She: *I can't.*

Me: *Think of something in the past that made you feel lonely or sorry for yourself, upset and rejected.*

She: *I can't.*

Me: *Think about the earliest time in your life when you experienced loneliness.*

She: *I can't.*

Me: (Talking to get some emotion going and tapping with Joan all the while …)

There is no end to my grief.
No one has suffered as much as me over
my grandmother's death.
Grieve me.
I'm so lonely.
Everyone should suffer as much as me.
Let me tell you how much I have suffered.
I want everyone to know the loneliness I felt at her death.
All the things I had to face.
All the poor me.
I'm the victim here.
My mother ignored me.
She was wrapped up in her own drama and she ignored me.
My mother ignored me and for that reason I am all alone
and I can never be happy.
I'm never going to let myself be happy ever again.
I'm going to seek solace in food and make myself fat.
I am going to punish myself with food.
I am going to punish my mother by stuffing my face with food.
That'll show her.
I'm going to get the comfort from food that I never got from
my mother.
Because she ignored me it proves I'm unlovable.
Clear it.
Clear it.
Clear it.

There was more to it than that and before we were done several other issues popped up and needed to be addressed.

But you get the idea. Although loneliness was a constant in her life; she was unable to bring herself to summon up the *emotion of loneliness* in order to work on it on her own.

Without the ability to get back into her familiar trance of loneliness we would never have succeeded in breaking through to create positive change.

Get the Most out of Your Tapping Efforts:

One approach to breaking through resistance is to come into your own power through *refusing to allow yourself to feel the emotion:*

Say, while tapping:

I refuse *to allow myself to feel (underlying emotion) in spite of the cost to myself.*

I refuse *to allow myself to feel whatever the emotion is until I feel perfectly safe doing so.*

See how that works for you!

Reason #12:

We Don't Get That We're the Cause of Our Own Distress

I don't know if this is true of you, but it's not so easy for most of us to accept the current wisdom that we are the source of our own problems and our own distress.

We also don't have a way to distinguish between what we are producing on our own, what we took on as labels, and what is other people's noise.

For some, it's overwhelming to think that we are fully responsible for our own lives. It's easier to blame family members, co-workers, our childhood, or outside circumstances for our stress. Facing up to this is not an easy task for most people. It wasn't for me.

This does not imply that we are guilty in any way. We always did the best we could with the emotional resources available to us at the time. And we are certainly not to blame for damage done to us in childhood.

Even so, we are the only ones who can do anything about it now that we are adults. Blaming anyone will not change our situation. It won't bring more fun into our life or life to our days.

Of course, the flip side to all this is empowerment. If I'm the cause, then it's in my control, and I have the power to change what I don't like about my life.

GET THE MOST OUT OF YOUR TAPPING EFFORTS

If the suggestion that you may be the cause of your own stress and distress ticks you off, you might want to get that out of your system. The first thing you want to tap on might be:

How dare you suggest I'm the cause of my own stress!

Reason #13:

There's Never Just One Cockroach

If there is a negative situation in our life, we may think: "If I fix that one thing, everything in my life will be better." That may work with someone who has had a rather easy life.

But, for many of us, it's not the whole story. You clean up one thing and another shows up. There's always more.

Once we have lowered the level of emotional intensity with tapping, another memory may bubble up that you might never guess would be connected. Of course, the connection is emotional and can be triggered by almost anything: a word, a thought, a look, a question, a smell, a physical sensation.

I have on videotape a session with "Annie" who felt that she made everyone more important than herself.

I ask her, "*If we were to compare your weight situation with a forest made up of trees and if you had to put a name to the trees in your 'weight forest' what name would you give it?*"

Annie says: "*Deprived.*" You can't help but notice how the word just comes through, without effort on her part. It's right there. Waiting to be expressed, even though it comes to her as a total surprise.

I say to her, "*Is there any part of your life where you feel deprived?*"

That brings up a well of emotion and she says,

> *Oh no, I'm going to cry.*
> *I'm deprived of doing things I want to do.*
> *My appetite came after I quit smoking.*
> *I'm drinking too much.*
> *I don't take care of myself.*

When we're working on the emotion of "feeling deprived" and we have it down to a "very low 2 – 3," her emotional intensity shoots right back up to a 10 as soon as we mention family.

She: *I was the 7th of 8 kids. There wasn't much attention given to me.*

Me: *And that made you feel …*

She: *Unloved.*

The emotional intensity increases as the emotion of feeling unloved surfaces to be cleared.

Then we have to deal with the sorrow ("*I didn't even know I had sorrow. That was new!*")

Then Annie has a hard time letting go of the sadness.

Deprived. Unloved. Sorrowful. Sad.

You work on one emotion, get it almost resolved, and something else comes up to be cleared. Even when you didn't realize that certain emotions were lurking beneath the surface.

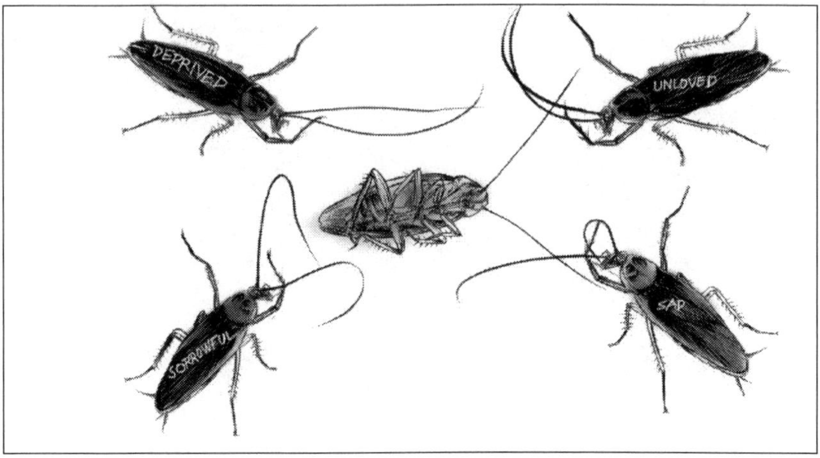

EMOTIONAL LITTLE DANCE

Finally, Annie comes to the realization that it's because of these interconnected but submerged emotions that she isn't taking the time to care for herself.

BREAKTHROUGH

There's an unexpected sequel to Annie's story which she revealed to me several weeks later. She had come to me to work on her weight but the big result was not weight loss. She said it was a breakthrough in her spirituality.

Get rid of the cockroaches and who knows what wealth is in store for you.

GET THE MOST OUT OF YOUR TAPPING EFFORTS

Approach the tapping from the standpoint of curiosity in what might be lurking under the surface. Do some "detective work" as Gary Craig would say.

If you don't care for the image of cockroaches, think in terms of something less obnoxious. In any case, your own metaphor will be far more powerful.

Reason #14:

We Are Limited by Deeply Held Beliefs Which Filter Our Experience and Thwart Our Progress

A BELIEF IS ONLY A THOUGHT YOU
CONTINUE TO THINK; AND WHEN YOUR
BELIEFS MATCH YOUR DESIRES, THEN YOUR DESIRES
MUST BECOME YOUR REALITY.

Abraham

Unexamined Beliefs

Our belief systems are often unconscious. That's why we're not aware of their existence. (It only makes sense that if we were aware, they would be conscious, right?)

Or they're so familiar to us that we're blind to them. We've lived with them for so long and they are such a part of us, we don't challenge their validity or usefulness.

Unless another person challenges or guides us around these beliefs, we continue to view and experience life through the same filters that created them. You know how effective that is at creating change, don't you?

A Sampling of Beliefs That Impede Our Progress

Religious Dogma

One client expressed the fear that tapping was in conflict with her faith. Another said, "Tapping is the devil's work. I worry that I'm taking matters into my own hands a little too much."

Money Messages

- "Do you think I'm made of money?"
  [Did you hear that one when you were a little kid?]

- "It's wrong to have money. It's wrong to be rich."

- "It's noble to be poor. Poor people are better than rich people."

- "You can't have money and be a good person at the same time."

- "Wanting more and asking for more is wrong, greedy and selfish."

- "I'm broke." [Now there's a powerful metaphor!]

- "Money is hard to come by."

- "It's wrong to get it too easily." [In other words, "I shouldn't be adequately rewarded for my natural talents and abilities," for one example.]

- "If I make a lot of money I am depriving someone else."

- "If I have money then people will make demands on me."

- Yada yada yada …

Here are some religious ones, for good measure:

- "The love of money is the root of all evil."
  [Often misquoted as "Money is the root of all evil."]

- "Rich people can never enter the Kingdom of Heaven."

- "It's harder to get a camel through the eye of a needle than for a wealthy man to get into heaven."

[Well, that about takes care of the philanthropists of this world.]

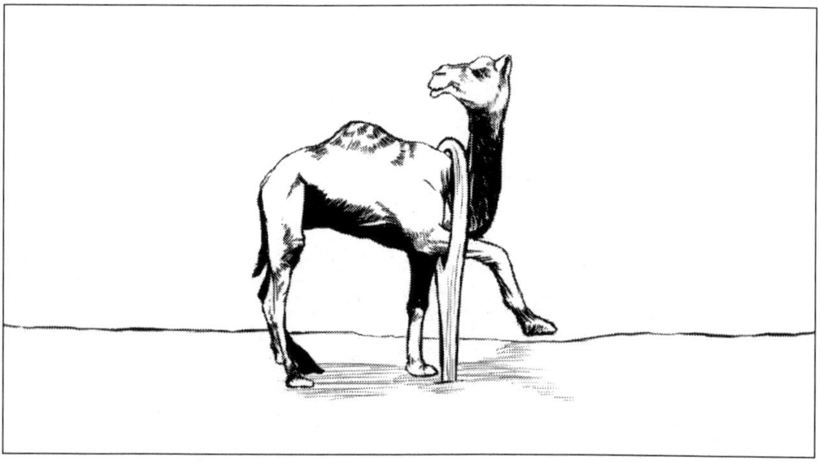

"IT'S HARDER TO GET A CAMEL THROUGH THE EYE OF A NEEDLE THAN FOR A WEALTHY MAN TO GET INTO HEAVEN."

And my own personal favorites, judging by the role I have allowed them to play in my life:

- "Life is about struggle and suffering."
- "You have to work hard for money."

I took these beliefs to mean that I had no value unless I struggled, suffered and worked hard. Those imprints still affect my life in devious ways in spite of the fact that I know there is no basis of truth to them.

> *If you believe that you must work hard in order to deserve the money that comes to you, then money cannot come to you unless you do work hard. Financial success, or any other kind of success, does not require hard work. It does require alignment of thought. You simply cannot offer negative thought about things that you desire and then make up for it with action or hard work. When you learn to direct your own thoughts, you will discover the true leverage of Energy alignment.*

ABRAHAM [VII]

A World of Hurt

I am working now with a 29-year old woman who just wants to be happy. She believes with all her heart that her miserable childhood is the cause of her life of discontent. She is beautiful, intelligent, vivacious, creative and many other delicious adjectives. She is well-educated and has an excellent job. An adoring and tolerant husband. Parents who have stuck by her through thick and thin. She informs me that she lives in a gorgeous contemporary home.

But she is filled with rage, resentment and lack of respect for people who had an easy childhood.

She actually feels superior to those who in her view of the world have suffered less than she has.

I thought, and then regretted telling her, that if we were to compare her early life experiences with those of my clients who in their early years were physically, mentally and emotionally abused, not to mention sexually molested, she would have no justification for her feelings of superiority.

She also would have no justification for her outbursts of rage if she gave up her belief: "*No one has suffered more than me.*"

When a lifetime has been built on negative positions, change may take a while.

SELF-IMAGE DOUBLE BINDS

- I worked with a woman who had the belief that "*I have to be perfect if I am going to have someone love me.*" She also realized "*... but by being perfect I intimidate people and drive them away.*"

- More recently, I had a few sessions with a young woman whom I consider to be absolutely gorgeous in a Barbie Doll kind of way. One of her life themes was loneliness. She was absolutely fixated on her image of beauty, spending all discretionary income on her appearance, and yet she complained of having no female friends because they were intimidated by her.

- A tall, blond woman said, "*I want to be slim and gorgeous but if I'm slim and gorgeous I won't have any friends because they'll all be jealous of me."* (In Reason #16: The secondary gains of having a problem outweigh the benefits of resolving the problem, I outline many of the underlying beliefs that can stand in the way of our progress in losing weight.)

- A highly intelligent client who said she had been an overly sensitive child told me, *"If I succeed in life I'm betraying my brother (who has a learning disability). If I fail I'm betraying my mom's hopes for me."*

- Until challenged, many men and women I've worked with carried the belief that they were responsible for everything and everyone around them. (*"I'm a good person because I worry. When I worry I show my family I love them."*) They would sacrifice and sabotage their own happiness in order to feel that they were a good person.

Now these are all very clear illustrations of what Gestalt Therapy labeled a "double bind." Damned if you do and damned if you don't. There's no way out.

You can see, can't you, that this sort of belief can keep you locked in place?

It's one reason "The Secret" doesn't work for most people, in spite of visualizations and affirmations and stating positive intentions. If an underlying belief is in contradiction to what we say we desire it will scuttle our best efforts.

I'm so Exceptional

You may have an underlying belief that tapping won't work for you. That you're a tough cookie. Beyond help. The exception to the rule. *"This is not going to work for me because I am an expert at stopping anything working for me."*

If we have the belief that a methodology isn't going to work because nothing else has ever worked, or that we're beyond help, or that we don't deserve to be well or happy, then we're not going to get the results we say we want.

Now why would this happen?

WHEN TAPPING DOESN'T WORK

You've no doubt heard of the Nocebo Effect—negative expectations resulting in negative outcomes? It is the diametric opposite to the Placebo Effect.

If we approach from a position that tapping won't work there's a good chance we will make that a self-fulfilling prophecy. Because the mind will do everything in its power to prove us right.

> *We have an innate ability to heal. That is what the placebo effect is all about.*
>
> *If the brain expects that a treatment will work, it sends healing chemicals into the bloodstream, which facilitates that. And the opposite is equally true and equally powerful: When the brain expects that a therapy will not work, it doesn't. It's called the 'nocebo' effect."*
>
> BRUCE H. LIPTON, PH.D., AUTHOR, THE BIOLOGY OF BELIEF

Deep, positive change requires clearing out every thought and belief that does not take us where we want to go.

For some of us, questioning whether a negative belief is getting in the way might just be the place to start.

I have no idea who said or wrote these words, but I find so much wisdom here:

> *The work you must do is not think positively about getting what you want but work diligently on all doubt that you will.*

Get the Most out of Your Tapping Efforts

If you find you have a belief that is getting in the way of your happiness you may find helpful some videos on my website. In the one titled "If I'm Not Sacrificing I'm Not A Good Person," you will see the sort of process we used to dissolve to zero – in six minutes flat – the belief "I fear I'm not a good person if I don't help other people." http://TappingTransformYourWorld.com/videos/

REASON #15:

WE ARE INFLUENCED BY DEEP-ROOTED SOCIETAL DOGMAS

SOCIETY EXPECTS A certain amount of grieving after the death of a loved one.

But how much is enough?

Some years ago, I had the privilege t-o work with a lovely woman, "Caroline," whose 20-year-old son had been fatally shot by an off-duty deputy sheriff during a prank gone wrong.

A mutual friend told me she had aged 10 years in the weeks since her son's death. I felt she had suffered long enough and offered to help take away some of her pain.

As you can imagine there were tears, intense grief and anger to resolve in our first session which lasted two and a half hours.

We tapped away the anger and grief and replaced the intrusive image in her mind of her son being shot to death with a favorite, sweet memory of him as a young boy. As she is a deeply religious person, she chose to have her son transmute to a guardian angel who would look after her forever.[1]

When she left was happy and calm.

A few days later, Caroline called me in anguish. She said she felt much better and had only cried once since our session. ("*Before that, it was all the time.*"). But a new concern was weighing heavily on her heart:

She: *I feel like I've lost my emotions.*

Me: *What do you mean when you say you have lost your emotions?*

She: *I mean I don't feel anything anymore.*

Me: *When you think about your older daughter, do you feel love?*

She: *Yes.*

Me: *When you think about your younger daughter, do you feel love*

She: *Yes.*

Me: *Do you feel love for your husband?*

She: *Yes.*

Me: *And when you think about (late son's name), do you feel love?*

She: *Yes.*

1 I think it important that a practitioner work within the client's belief system regardless whether that belief is shared.

Me: *So you still feel the emotion of love?*

She: *Yes.*

Me: *So when you say you aren't feeling emotions, do you mean you're not feeling the negative emotions?*

She: *Yes.*

Me: *And is that a bad thing?*

She: *Yes. This week I attended another meeting at my church for bereaved mothers and fathers. This time, as everyone went around the room introducing themselves and talking about what brought us there, I was the only one who didn't cry. Some of them had lost a son or daughter as long as 16 or 17 years ago and they were crying as though it had just happened. I was at peace with (my son's) death.*

Me: *And?*

She: *I felt they were judging me.*

You know where this is going, don't you?

We had to work through her guilt at not wasting the rest of her life in grief, the way these other loving, bereft parents were doing.

Unlike them, she had re-imprinted the tragedy with memories of love. Her son was now her protector. She was living in the moment again and able to be fully present with her husband, daughters, parents and extended family.

We then had to deal with her dejection at no longer feeling a part of this group of people who had shaped their lives around the unbearable loss of a child.

GET THE MOST OUT OF YOUR TAPPING EFFORTS

If you are still grieving the loss of a loved one and it is affecting other aspects of your life in a negative way, and you want to be happy again, you might want to ask yourself these questions and tap on any emotions that arise:

- How long do I have to grieve to prove my love?
- Does my grief make anything better? Does it change anything?
- Do I believe I will be judged by others if I don't grieve long enough?
- Does that grief make any difference now to the person I am grieving?
- Or am I grieving for myself?
- If I stop grieving and instead remember my loved one with joyful memories will that hurt him in any way? Or is she in a better place now?

Reason #16:

The Secondary Gains of Having a Problem Outweigh the Benefits of Resolving the Problem

In the first two years of my tapping practice, I discovered that it was easier for most of my clients to overcome trauma, even early childhood trauma, than it was to lose weight.

Strange, I thought. Why is that?

I think it's because with trauma you *know* there's a problem. With trauma, at every level of your being, you know that something is not right. Your system welcomes the release.

But for issues other than trauma, sometimes there are very powerful emotional reasons for hanging on. Take weight, for example.

You may associate food with love. Or the weight may be keeping you safe in some way. Perhaps it's a way to avoid rejection. Or intimacy. Whatever. That sets up a natural resistance.

If the secondary gains or secret advantages outweigh the desired solution, change ain't never gonna happen.

For these reasons I will not work with a person when a physical injury lawsuit with potential financial payoff is pending. I know from personal experience that it works against all legal advice to take any action to mitigate the pain. Sadly, I also know that the pain continues to intensify under these conditions.

The same applies when the person with Fibromyalgia balks at the idea of giving up their social security disability. The underlying reason for not getting better is just too strong.

WHAT DO I REALLY WANT?

When I first began my EFT practice, I worked with a strikingly beautiful professional woman with a serious weight problem. (Her judgment.) On the surface, "Jill" was desperate to lose 47 pounds. (Not fifty pounds. Forty-seven pounds.)

We had resolved all her relationship and betrayal and self-concept issues. But still the weight didn't budge.

I asked Jill what she thought would happen if she were slim? Was there any negative aspect to losing the weight?

At first, she couldn't see any advantages to maintaining her present situation.

With prodding, she responded …

- *If I was slim I would draw more attention. As an overweight person I'm not as visible.*

- *I would not fit in with women my age. If I was tall and slim and blond ... women don't like women who are tall and slim and blond.* (Hmm, I thought, now there's a belief system.)

- *Potential customers won't confide in me. Other people who are heavy tend to talk to you more easily. The common thread of weight wouldn't be there. Camaraderie would be broken.*

- *I would have to watch what I eat to maintain the weight loss. I don't want to have to constantly work hard on my weight. Now I can indulge versus working hard and always having to be aware of my food intake.*

- *People would see me as having it all together. A successful business woman. Always happy. People think beautiful people have no problems. That life is easier for them. I don't want people to think I have life easy.*

- *People will have higher expectations of you. Maybe people are jealous of you.*

- *I have to be overweight in order to be accepted by my peers.*

- *I worry that my skin is going to be all flabby if I lose weight.* (Well, okay. She may have something there if she waits until she is in her late 50's to give it a whirl.)

And, finally, she admitted the big one:

- *I love to go out with friends, drink beer and eat fatty foods. The social piece is more important to me than my weight and my health.*

The needs for inclusion, acceptance and anonymity in a crowd were more powerful than the desire to lose weight.

These were all issues Jill had never openly admitted to herself. On her own, do you think she would ever have gotten to the origin of her weight issue with these powerful reasons for holding on to her excess pounds?

Not too likely.

You can guess which way things went, can't you?

Jill chose the camaraderie of friends who love to toy with the idea of losing weight. But who never will.

Get the Most out of Your Tapping Efforts

Moment of Truth

Ask yourself:

> *Are there any secret advantages to maintaining the status quo?*
> *What do I get out of it?*
> *Is there any negative aspect to clearing the issue?*
> *What do I lose if I let this go?*
> *Will I be safe?*
> *Do I even want to let this go?*

Reason #17:

We Fail to Connect the Dots

Ring the bells that still can ring
Forget your perfect offering
There is a crack in everything
That's how the light gets in.

Leonard Cohen, 1934 – 2016

Often, we're spinning our wheels and unable to make the connections between what happened in our past and what is going on with us in the present. I'm not sure, but that may be especially true of those of us who grew up in a family that wasn't your run-of-the-mill dysfunctional.

Sometimes the trauma happened so early or so consistently in our lives that we don't have perspective. We don't give it the importance it deserves when we're working on our own.

That's because we tend to normalize things. What I mean by that is we're so used to living with situations, we're so used to the patterns in our own life, that we believe they're "normal."

Family Secrets

Let me tell you a story that – up to now – I have only ever told to one or two close friends.

I grew up in what appeared to be a happy household. My mother was a stay-at-home mom. From the time I was eight I went to a convent school and wore the unloveliest black-uniform you ever did see. We looked like little nuns chicks with our stiff, starched white collar and cuffs. When not in uniform, I wore little dresses with pretty, starched pinafores.

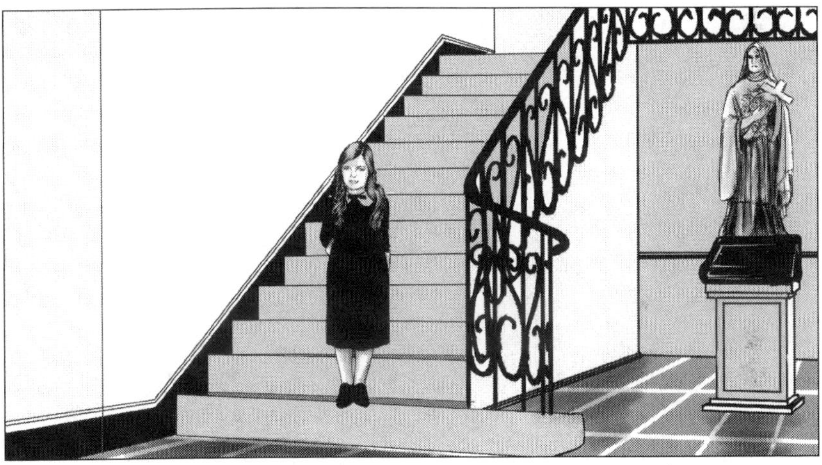

My older sister and I studied music and dance and were expected to make our parents proud. My mother and father never went beyond grades 6 and 9, respectively, but that was beside the point. They expected us to excel in school and all our activities.

That was the surface stuff. My early and teen years were marred by family violence and threats of violence.

I had an angry, alcoholic father who in a drunken rage would storm into the bedroom I shared with my sister and threaten that he was going to get a gun, kill our mother and then kill us in our sleep.

I was afraid to fall asleep at night because I had to stay alert. Just in case.

Sleepless in …

You can just imagine the havoc this played with my sleep patterns over the years. Always on the alert. Always awake at the slightest sound.

I believed him. My older sister didn't. She would say, "Oh go to sleep. He won't kill us. He's too afraid of the police."

(Such is the power of belief. It has made all the difference in our lives. She has always been able to shrug things off and sleep soundly while, until recently, I often hovered on the edge of sleep.)

A practitioner who knows my story said to me, "Even though you understood as an adult that it wasn't normal to live in a household where your life was constantly being threatened you never questioned that the feeling that your life was always in danger could be directly related to your insomnia. You were surprised when we made the connection just now."

As my story illustrates, we don't always draw the lines on our own.

That's why even seasoned practitioners seek each other out when they hit rough spots as part of their commitment to continuous personal growth. A third party brings a fresh perspective and helps us draw the lines.

Reason #18:

An Unacknowledged Emotion Is Holding Everything Firmly in Place

If you are still struggling with something that happened years ago, in spite of having seen therapists for decades, you can be sure that you have not got to the source.

I worked with a woman whose husband had been killed in an industrial accident decades earlier. She had never fully recovered from his death and it was still affecting her daily life.

She felt she had never sufficiently grieved his death, in spite of years of grief counselling, cognitive psycho-therapy, and prescription drugs.

It became clear to me that sorrow and grief were only part of her ongoing suffering.

Anger

At the heart of her misery was that she had never acknowledged to herself or to anyone how *angry* she was at her husband for dying and leaving her to raise a toddler and an unborn child on her own. In her mind, it wasn't acceptable to be angry with the man she loved who was no longer alive and could not defend himself. It wasn't nice. It wasn't rational. Friends and family would judge her harshly. The anger had to be suppressed.

We tapped to zero all feelings of anger, rage, impotent rage, betrayal, blame, shame at having these emotions, forgiveness, and whatever else bubbled to the surface to be cleared.

She contacted me two days later to say she felt calm. Her life had changed. Family members were treating her better. (That's one of the virtues of doing this work: when we change at a deep, fundamental level, the people around us change. Everything in our universe begins to transform. It's a tangible sign that, in every moment, we are creating our own reality.)

> *As above, so below, as within, so without,*
> *as the universe, so the soul ...*
>
> HERMES TRISMEGISTUS

If you're like me, you'll probably want another example, or two ...

GUILT

I once worked with a woman who had severe PTSD. She had years earlier been involved in a horrendous encounter in which several people had died. Our breakthrough came when she finally acknowledged the guilt she felt at the angry words she had spoken to one of the victims just before her death.

Shame

I worked with a severely depressed woman who could not hold down a job and who, in her early 40s, was still financially dependent on her parents. The consensus of several therapists, she said, was that she was still suffering from having been sexually molested at an early age by her late uncle.

Turns out, the underlying issue was not that she had been "diddled with" (as she put it) but that she had *enjoyed being diddled with*. She loved her uncle, she loved the gifts and the attention, she loved that the two of them had their own little secret, and she loved the sensuality of their encounters, even at a very young age. She had never admitted this to anyone. She had played along with various therapists' attempts to help her because she felt her true sexual response was unacceptable.

I have found that the secret to diffusing the effects of traumatic life events is to get to the *invisible, underlying, often unacknowledged emotion that is the root cause of a person's suffering.*

A study of post-traumatic stress experienced by people who were involved in military combat bears this out:

> *The idea of "moral injury" as a cause of PTSD is new to psychiatry. The American Psychiatric Association is only now considering new diagnostic criteria for the disorder that would include feelings of shame and guilt ...*

Gregg Zoroya, "Study suggests feelings of guilt are a top PSTD cause," USA TODAY International Edition, 28 November, 2011

If you suspect that you or someone you love may be suffering from this scourge, the PTSD Foundation of America has on its website a thorough Self-Assessment Test. http://ptsdusa.org/what-is-ptsd/get-help/

I would not suggest that anyone attempt to tap on traumatic memories of war atrocities, natural disasters, terrorist events, mass violence or serious accidents on their own.

Since it can be too painful and possibly create deeper issues to tap on certain deep emotional content on one's own I would suggest working with a practitioner who has specialized training in dealing with trauma.

REASON #19:

WE DON'T RECOGNIZE THE VALUABLE CLUES FROM OUR OWN MIND'S METAPHORS

THE METAPHOR IS PROBABLY
THE MOST FERTILE POWER POSSESSED BY MAN.

José Ortega y Gasset,
Philosopher & Essayist 1883 – 1955

METAPHORS ARE A creative and tangible way of expressing a mental or feeling state. The use of visual images makes it possible to break through to deeper emotions. When metaphors are very specific to the individual they can be a powerful healing tool.

One of my favorite metaphorical images sprang to life as "Joan" and I were working on her experience of grief.

As so often happens, we were tapping on one emotion when another surfaced, demanding attention.

Raven of Grief

Joan said: *"I let grief be really big in my life. It feels like a weight in my chest. It sits in my neck like a huge black 300-pound raven just sitting there and it won't get off."*

I had her talk to the raven while tapping, stream of consciousness style. I told her to just say whatever came into her head.

She: *I'm never going to let you go. Never. Because you give me a reason for living. You define me. And here's what I love about you: with you on my chest I don't have to pick a direction.*

You're a good excuse to stop me from moving forward. [Now there's an insight!]

Me: *What does having a heavy 300-pound raven sitting on your chest prevent you from doing?*

She: *I can't get up and get on with my life. I can't decide what makes me happy. I can't go through with a direction. So maybe I'm afraid. Maybe he holds me back so I don't have to act.*

Oh, my gosh! It's really me doing it to me. [Another insight.]

Me: *Thank you bird.*

She: *Thank you bird.*

Me: *Does he have a name?*

She: *Big-a**ed Bird.* [Lots of laughter]

Me: *So, Big-a**ed Bird, thank you for everything you do for me.*

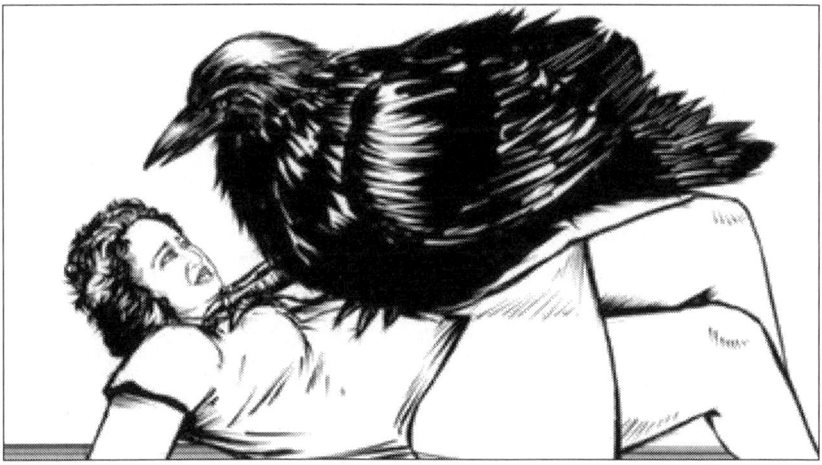

Raven of Grief

She: *Thank you for keeping me safe. In one place. Keeping me from knowing myself. Thank you for the excuse. Thanks for the memories.* [Laughter] *You have been really, really useful, Bird. Look what you've done for me all these years. You keep me from moving forward. You provide the perfect excuse to not take charge of my life. I think you're the most beautiful bird, you're big and you've got a great big a**.*

Me: *What is Big-a**ed Bird doing now?*

She: *He's sitting doing nothing, just holding me down which is what I've been doing all year, holding myself back. So he's like a mirror. Thank you for being a mirror. Thank you for being my weight. Thank you for providing what I need to stay in place.*

> *The choking feeling gives me a health reason now for not getting on with my life.*

After we tapped on the choking feeling and the pressure on her chest from all that weight …

Me: *Does Big-a**ed Bird have something to say to you?*

She: *He turned to me and said, "Well, you never told me to get off."*

Me: *So why is he here?*

She: *I've been feeding him.*

Me: *How?*

She: *Literally, I fed him. That's how they stay. You feed them. I welcomed him.*

Me: *How long do you want him around?*

She: *I don't.*

Me: *But he loves you. How can you give up someone who loves you?*

She: *I'm going to tell him to get off. "Get off my chest."*

Me: *Does he?*

She: *He won't get off.*

Me: *Why won't he get off?*

She: *I think he thinks I need him.*

Me: *Do you?*

She: *I don't need him any more.*

Me: *He thought he was keeping you safe. Can you make him get smaller and smaller and smaller so that he fits into the palm of your hand?*

She: *He's getting smaller and smaller.*

Me: *When he gets tiny, throw him up into the sky. He can either go up and disappear into nothingness or he can choose to become a bright star. Or anything else you want.* [I didn't make notes on this part and can't remember what Joan chose to do with her Big-A**ed friend. But I doubt that he'll be back!]

She: *I'm trying to get used to not having this weight on my chest. Anyone would feel a sense of loss after all these years. I'm going to give myself 30 seconds.*

Me: *Give yourself as much time as you need. You don't need to feed the raven any more.*

She: *When I'm tempted to eat to comfort myself, am I feeding me or the raven?*

Me: *That's your raven. Only you know that. Only you can decide what role you're going to give him.*

One of the things I love about this story is Joan's realization that the bird is her own projection, her own creation.

She later wrote to me to say that working through the metaphor enabled her to finally find a direction and move on with her life.

> *I feel I got rid of some big chunks. I had this image before that you were going to help me peel things away. I feel good. Life is good. I'm just grateful. Thank you.*

And since I like the topic so much, here is another example of using visual images to break through to deeper emotions. In this instance, a series of images helped me and my client uncover, then dissolve, the true cause of her sadness.

Sadness as an Anchor

Me: *What does your sadness remind you of?*

She. *My sadness is like an anchor.*

Me: *Hold your anchor.*

She: *It's heavy. I can barely hold it. Its 50 lbs.*

Me: *It's yours. You've been carrying it around for 50 years. Can you make it heavier? 100 pounds maybe?*

She: *It's kind of who I am. It's the anchor or nothing.*

She: [Tapping]

> *Let go the resistance to letting go the familiar.*
> *Let go the attachment to my anchor.*
> *It keeps me safe.*
> *It protects me.*
> *I can't get too close to anyone when the anchor is in the way.*

Me: *Just for a moment, consider whether you can put it down.*

She: *Yeaaah. I want to let it go but I don't want to let it go. Safety. Fear. The familiar.*

Me: *Let go my anchor.*

She: *Let go my anger.* [Now there's a Freudian slip[2] if I ever heard one!]

She: *Let go this anger.*

Me: *That's all this is. Under the sadness is the anger.*

She: *Yes! Anger at life. Anger at the universe. Anger at God.*

Me: *Can you give your anger a shape?*

She: *Yes. It's Vesuvius, bursting in flames.*

Me: *What would happen if you let go this anchor … I mean, this anger?*

She: *If I let it go I'll be weak. If I use anger I'll have some sense of control because I don't know how to protect myself.*

Me: *How well is that working for you?*

She: *I use the anger to supposedly make me strong. I'll also lose my identity. I'd be vulnerable … in a place of not knowing. And that feels scary.*

Me: *And do you feel in control?*

She: *No.*

Me: *And do you want to feel in control?*

She: *Yes.*

2 You know what a Freudian slip is, don't you? You say one thing and mean your mother!

Me: *Are you open to the possibility of giving up your anger in order to feel in control?*

She: *I'm open to the possibility of giving up my anger.*

We tap on memories of childhood episodes when she felt required to suppress all emotion in order to feel safe within family rules.

Me: *What is happening with your anger now?*

She: *It's really small. The flames are just a little sputter and smoke.*

Me: *Now what?*

She: *I forgive myself for holding on to this powerless anger.*

The anchor morphs into Vesuvius bursting in flames and the anger dissipates in the form of a kite that she blows away with a gust of wind.

She: *Now I'm on the edge of the cliff, waving to everybody. I'm calm. Excited. Happy. There's a feeling of anticipation.*

Something else surfaces that needs to be dealt with:

She: *There's something else in my solar plexus. It's like a grey mist. I have the feeling that this can't last. It's a 5.*

Me: *Would you like to turn the grey mist into a glorious sunset?*

She: *Let it become something beautiful in my life. There's a little puffy cloud and that makes me enjoy the blue sky even more.*

We tap on the feeling that this can't last. And then, up pops another image:

She: *Sadness is like a balloon in me.*

Tapping:

She: *I just love my sadness. I am so attached to my sadness.*

Me: *Like a child with a balloon?*

She: *I built a whole life around this?*

Me: *It's your balloon. You can choose to decide how long to hang on to it.*

She: *It's outside of me now. The balloon is yellow. I let it all go into that blue sky. It could become the sun.*

> *I can create my own sunshine.*
> *That's what I'm doing today.*
> *I can live in sunshine.*
> *I can let myself really enjoy my job.*
> *I can let myself appreciate that I have work that keeps me from being bored.*
> *I am free to be myself.*
> *I am free to create calm in my life.*
> *And that's my choice.*

Me: *Where are you now?*

She: *I'm calm.*

Me: *Where's your sadness now?*

She: *What sadness?*

At our next session, the anger and sadness were out of her system.

GET THE MOST OUT OF YOUR TAPPING EFFORTS

The power of the metaphor is that it speaks to the individual. If you like the idea of working with your own metaphors, here's a place to start:

> *"What does this remind me of?"*

What does your current problem or feeling or mental state remind you of? If you were to represent it as a vivid image, what would that image be?

Play with it, speak to it, and tap as you follow the chain of emotions and meanings, allowing the images to morph and take you wherever they want to go.

Reason #20:

The Thing We Say We Want Is a Threat to Our Identity

THE ONLY THING KEEPING YOU FROM WHAT YOU WANT IS YOUR STORY ABOUT WHY YOU CAN'T HAVE IT.

Tony Robbins

SOMETIMES WE'RE SO addicted to our own narrative that we've created an identity with it. So it can be hard to give up our story.

Several years ago, I worked with a woman, "Kim", who ten years previously had been involved in a horrific, high-profile, multi-car crash on a major highway.

As so often happens, she developed Post-Traumatic Stress Disorder (PTSD) and was treated by a psychiatrist for many years.

After the crash, Kim's life took on new meaning. She left her high-profile profession and became an advocate for people who suffer from PTSD.

Kim told me she had spent tens of thousands of dollars on her recovery but still had panic attacks when driving on the highway. She experienced flashbacks even when driving in the city whenever cars lined up bumper-to-bumper waiting for the light to turn green.

She was still unable to look at photos that had been published by the press. The 10th anniversary of the crash was in sight and the newspapers would be calling on her again for her comments. Kim couldn't face the thought and it was causing her a great deal of stress.

I invited her to a complimentary EFT session. Without going into specifics here, we worked through Gary Craig's Tell The Story Technique. We cleared some profound emotions surrounding the accident: terror, horror and previously unacknowledged anger and guilt.

Part way through our session, she marveled: "*I am saying 'I am safe now' ... that's a breakthrough already.*"

At the end of our two hours she could recount every detail of the accident without any emotional trigger. She said, "*It's really amazing. I see everything lighter, brighter. Wow! It's like putting years of therapy into one session.*"

When Kim left my office she looked radiant, visibly ten years younger in appearance. I told her to call me should anything come up because we had done some deep work. If something came up we would handle it over the phone or have her return to my office.

She did not call as promised. Much to my surprise she did not book another session, as she had said she would, to clear other matters.

Weeks later, over dinner at which I was a guest at her home, Kim declared, with quite a bit of passion, that EFT might work for weight loss but it wasn't powerful enough to work for PTSD because the night of our session she had gone home and "abused" her husband. [I didn't ask.]

I was gob-smacked.

Words failed me. Had I my wits about me, I might have said, "*Well, going home and abusing your husband for the first time ever sounds like a pretty powerful result to me. You had an abreaction.*"

Alas, I missed the moment.

After dinner, she invited me and her other guest to see her brand new Mac. On the super-sized monitor was the 10th anniversary pictorial history of the horrific event, as recently published in the local newspaper.

There was no show of emotion. She spoke calmly. She might have been talking about a newspaper article she had read that in no way involved her personally.

Who wouldn't call that progress?

Again, I was so stunned I missed the moment.

This is a prime example of what Dr. Roger Callahan called The Apex Problem. Sometimes the shift a person experiences is so profound that it's as if they never had the problem in the first place.

And sometimes a person's identity is so caught up in their story that they may not be willing to acknowledge the extent of positive change that has taken place.

They may also reject the change because they have embraced something that happened to them as integral part of their self-image. When it is gone, they aren't quite sure how to cope.

Reason #21:

We Got Hijacked by the Beliefs of a Child

Of course, we are all children (even though some of us have developed a few wrinkles ...)

Gary Craig, Founder,
Emotional Freedom Techniques (EFT)

We tend to think of trauma in terms of major life events that we experienced in our early, teen or adult years: an accident, a physical assault, even forgetting our lines on opening night of our high school play.

But we forget that trauma is a matter of perception. To a small child, an older brother throwing a favorite teddy bear out the window in teasing jest may be perceived and held in the body as a trauma.

For that reason, our lives are often shaped by conclusions we drew before the age of reason, as we were forming our identity and before we had a perspective on life.

Sometimes we have difficulty getting tapping results on our own because we're not aware that we're still held in place by beliefs we took on as a young child.

Here are a few examples from my files …

THE OMNIPOTENT CHILD

When I first put out my shingle as an EFT practitioner, I worked with a woman whose life themes were *"It's All My Fault."* | *"I'm Bad."* | *"I Hurt People."* | *"I'm Not Safe."* | *"People are not safe around me."* |*"I don't deserve to be happy."*

In spite of decades of talk therapy, "Felicity" was caught in a time warp. She had the body build of a frail child and the face of a mature, depressed, middle-aged woman.

Without going into the particulars of why she booked an appointment, it soon became clear that there was a connection between her current feelings of panic and her childlike belief that she was responsible for all the bad things that happened to people around her.

When she was 7 or 8 years old Felicity lived with and looked after a maiden aunt and uncle. They lived on a farm.

In Felicity's story, she was responsible for cooking and cleaning and otherwise running the household. (Whether or not a child this age is even capable of these tasks is immaterial because we are working within a person's own beliefs, memories and perceptions. It does not matter that time may have distorted the facts.)

Her uncle worked in the fields. His sister, the aunt, had rheumatoid arthritis and was confined to a wheelchair. She was not all that nice a person, from what I was hearing. And she seemed to expect an awful lot of a seven-year-old. This aunt *"lost most of her life because she couldn't walk and she was in pain and that makes you grumpy."*

She would tell young Felicity, "*You'll be the death of me.*"

One day the aunt's self-fulfilling prophecy came to pass. Felicity was not able to help her in her last moments.

> *She was on the sofa and she told me to call 911. I froze in panic and was unable to pick up the phone. When she died, her eyes were staring at me. It looked to me like she was saying, 'See, I told you.' She always said I wasn't old enough to be helpful and one of these days something would happen and she would die because of me.*

Felicity believed, as only a young child can believe, that she was personally responsible for her aunt's death. Therefore, she deserved to be punished. For the rest of her life, apparently.

I didn't see this at first. Only later in the session did it become evident that I was dealing, not with an adult, but with a person who was frozen in time. Her words reflected the mindset of a 7-year-old: "*It's all my fault. People around me get hurt. I'm not safe to be around. I'm a bad person.*"

Through tears she told me, "*When you tell me I'm a good person I just want to throw up.*"

"Held Hostage by a 7-Year Old"

Near the end of our time together, she had a golden insight: "*I feel like I'm being held hostage by a 7-year old.*"

But when she left that first session I knew that, in spite of that insight, no significant change had taken place. She now had some perspective on the situation but we still had not broken through to the core.

Inspiration hit overnight. I thought, if I'm dealing with a 7-year old I need to approach this differently. So I called and asked her to come back the next day for a tapping session with her 7-year old self.

I tapped on her as an adult and she tapped on herself as a child:

> *I killed my aunt.*
> *I kill people.*
> *Nobody is safe around me.*
> *I'm bad.*
> *I'm irresponsible.*
> *I deserve to be punished.*

Now we were getting somewhere.

After many tearful rounds, focusing on severe emotions, I was communicating with an adult.

At long last she began to see that it was safe to move on. If I had known about Matrix Reimprinting[viii] at the time, the session would have been that much more valuable for Felicity because we could have reimprinted this sinister episode with something joyful and transformed the core belief that had to date governed her life.

HIDDEN IMPACT

It is not always this easy to connect the dots.

Sometimes, a belief from childhood will have a profound impact on our adult lives in ways that appear unrelated to the original event.

Here is one such instance, in the words of my client "Ellen" …

We had a piano in our home when I was a child and taking lessons was my idea.

As a six years old, my idea of playing the piano was having fun, plunking at the keys with one hand and enjoying the sounds I created. My mother had her own concept of how I should be practicing. She was always scolding me from the kitchen, telling me that I wasn't doing it right. All this money was being wasted on me.

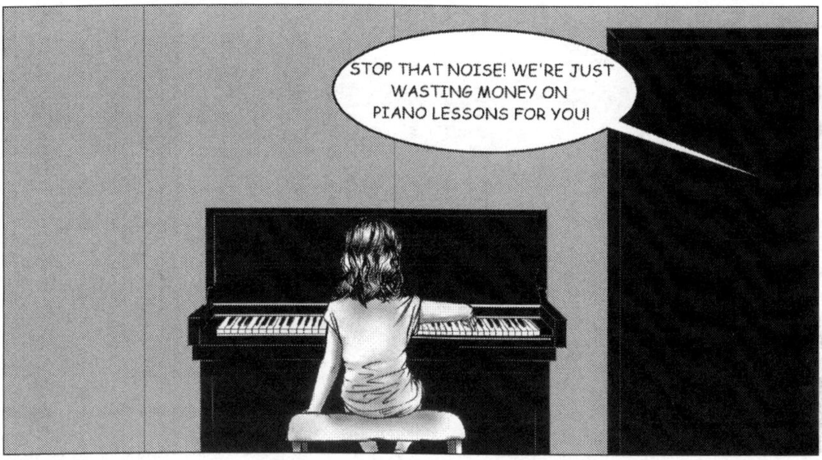
STOP THAT NOISE! WE'RE JUST WASTING MONEY ON PIANO LESSONS FOR YOU!

I felt so guilty. I stopped playing and quit my piano lessons, crushed at the thought that I was wasting my mother's money, wasting my father's money, and bankrupting the family.

From that experience grew the thought pattern: "You are not allowed to be joyful. You are unworthy. It's not your money and you have no right to it."

I have always had the feeling that I am not entitled to money, even to money I have earned myself. It's a feeling of powerlessness over money.

Now I see how the piano episode still shows up in my life today. As an artist, I can give my paintings away, but I can't put a price on them and sell them for what they are worth.

No amount of tapping will produce the desired result if we don't make the connection to the source of the belief.

TO BALANCE THINGS OFF A BIT ...

I'm including a few lighter clips from childhood that I think you'll enjoy. In each instance, we've taken painful situations that caused a lot of grief to my client all her life, released the negative emotion through tapping, and then reframed each episode into a humorous point of view.

YOU'RE NOT A COW. YOU'RE NOT A COW.

During a session, I was telling my assistant Amelia (her real name), about another client in her 30's whose *entire life* had been affected by the painful memory of her beloved Kindergarten teacher falsely accusing her of not putting away the scissors after a little group project. (True story.)

Amelia recalled her own calamitous episode with her Kindergarten teacher that had remained with her for over 30 years. The teacher had been giving lessons about barnyard animals and where food comes from. It was snack time and she was serving milk and cookies.

Me: *So, what happened?*

She: *I said, "You're like a cow. You're bringing us milk." I thought I was saying something smart.* [Pause] *I keep seeing her angry face."* [Tears]

Amelia rated her humiliation at the memory a 9 out of 10 on the intensity scale.

She: *I always thought I was such a stupid, bad child for saying that.*

We tapped on that for a few minutes and a more mature outlook broke through.

She: *How can such an insignificant little thing have such power over your life? It starts a pattern of making you feel bad. "Mrs. Low-Self-Esteem, I didn't mean to imply that you were fat like a cow. I forgive you. I forgive myself."*

Me: *You look back on it now is there any trigger?*

She: *No.*

Me: *What do you want to say to the little girl?*

She: *It's not important. Her low self-esteem has nothing to do with you. Just go play.*

Me: *Does she?*

She: *Yes. She's playing in the sandbox. She's happy now.*

Little Boys Can Be Such Brats!

Sometimes a playground incident can go too far— would you believe a lifetime for the same sweet Amelia?

Before we get into the dialogue I had with her I want to affirm that there is nothing funny about childhood bullying. Bullying is a serious problem (that) "throws a long shadow over affected people's lives.[ix]

Its victims "are more likely to suffer from poor health, loneliness, depression, unemployment, even substance abuse and attempts at suicide" than the remainder of the population.

I have worked with a number of victims of childhood bullying and most of those conversations did not involve laughter. Resolution. But no belly laughs. This one was an exception.

She: *I was laughed at in public school because I was poor. In line in the schoolyard, one of the boys made fun of me.*

Me: *What did he say?*

She: *He said, "What kind of an outfit is that?"*

Me: *That's enough to wreck anybody's life!*

She: [Laughing] *That's ridiculous. What have I done with that? I let it ruin my life.*

[Now there's a luscious insight that she had never been able to come to on her own without a third party reframing the whole episode.]

She: *He was a normal, sporty type.*

Me: *Let's call him Normie then.*

She: [Laughing] *On Planet Thrive that's what we call normal people who don't have our chemical sensitivities. Normies don't understand about perfume. I'm too sensitive for normies.*

Me: *Then that's the name we have to give the little brat. Normies are everywhere. They're crawling all over the place.*

Then we were convulsed with laughter.

She: *I have earned my status as a hypersensitive person.*

Me: *What do you want to say to Normie?*

She: *"Get away, squirt." That works. He was short. That's why he was bullying me. "You're short. Get over it!"*

Me: *What's the look on Normie's face?*

She: *Scorn. Mischievous. Mocking. Nasty.*

Tapping:

> *I forgive myself.*
> *I forgive Normie.*
> *He was just a kid.*
> *I was just a kid.*
> *It's all over now.*
> *Time to let it go.*
> *Blaming Normie for how I feel.*
> *He was probably just teasing me because I was so cute.*
> *I'm letting go of my problems.*
> *I forgive myself.*
> *I forgive him.*

Me: *Go back to your memory and look at your face. What do you see?*

She: *A light, detached, "well isn't that amusing" sort of expression. Normie shrank and I got bigger.*

Me: *Here comes Normie again, "What kind of an outfit is that?" Any trigger?*

She: *No. Oh my gawd, this is so hilarious. I think I'm at the beginning of a very significant healing process. Taking offense and letting something so insignificant go this far. I'm over it. My victimhood is leaving me.*

In Amelia's life, bullying had escalated into violent physical attacks and abusive relationships in her teenage and early adult years. We dealt with these episodes in later sessions that did not involve laughter.

What Amelia has learned is that while she is not at all responsible for what happened to her as a child, maintaining the role of victim and carrying the memory in one's heart and mind takes a lot of energy and does not make for a happy life.

Feeling the victim robs us of the freedom that comes from knowing we have choice.

Whatever happened in the past is over. It is we who continue to torture ourselves in the present and only we can bring that mental torture to an end.

Here's a story of another girl – one who could never quite measure up …

I Guess I'll Never Be a Ballerina

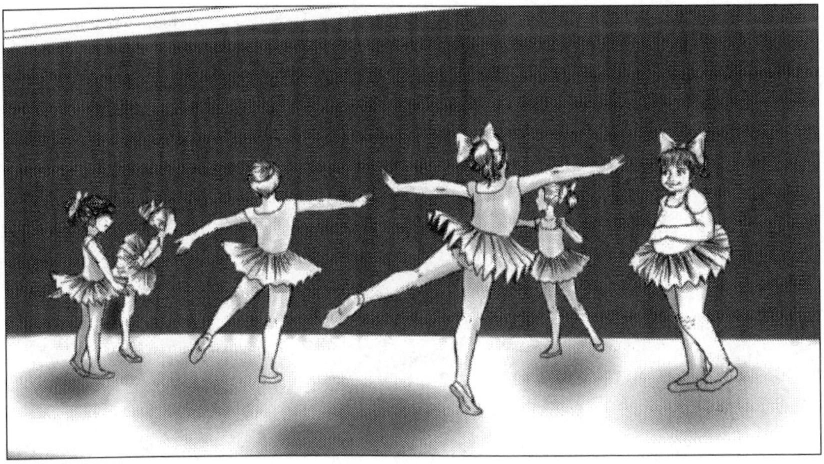

"Cheryl" had felt inadequate, judged and humiliated throughout her adult life.

She said: *"My mom signed me up for ballet when I was 6 or 7. My brother told me I looked like a little elephant thumping up on the stage."*

She made a decision that impacted her entire life: *"I'm inadequate because I'm not the ideal image. Being overweight is humiliating. Now it's like I'm proving them right. I'm living up to that image."*

We worked through the pain of the memory and then changed the scene in her mind, filling the stage with baby elephants dressed in tutus of various hues.

When I saw this client months later, she had lost the extra pounds.

I'M A BIG GIRL NOW

Sometimes, in our innocence and inexperience, we may have a distorted view of the meaning of a word.

A different client again, whose sisters were considerably older than she, always told her she was a big girl. She took this on as a negative label.

I pointed out to her that we always say to little kids, "*What a big girl!" "What a big boy!" and we mean it as a positive.*

She came to this realization: "*I grew up to be 200 lbs. because as a little child I misinterpreted what 'big girl' meant. I took on a negative image of myself. Now is the moment. I am taking back my full power.*"

NOT JUST BOYS CAN BE SUCH BRATS!

My older sister and I used to take pleasure in terrorizing our beautiful and much younger (and spoiled, we thought) sister. Younger sister tells me that one day we lifted her and dangled her by the legs upside down into a smelly outdoor garbage can. (We're all good friends now and all has been forgiven. I think! She did trust me enough to become one of my very first EFT tapping clients!)

When I told her I was thinking of including these goings-on in my book she jokingly said to tell you "it isn't something that crosses my mind, but it probably ruined my three marriages!"

Good questions to ask yourself:

- When in my childhood did I not feel safe?
- Have I allowed painful childhood episodes to define my life?
- Is any part of me being held hostage by my child self?
- Am I going to let an experience I had as a 5-, 7- or 9-year old define my life?
- What are the chances that an event from my childhood has morphed into another context and had a far deeper impact on my life than previously realized?

GET THE MOST OUT OF YOUR TAPPING EFFORTS

If you suspect that an early childhood belief is playing havoc with your happiness today, my best suggestion is to tap on your child self.

[Refer to Part III: Tap on your child self and 9-Step process to clear the structure of a problem.]

Reason #22:

The Story We Tell Ourselves Sabotages Our Best Efforts

Each and every component that makes up your life experience is drawn to you by the powerful Law of Attraction's response to the thoughts you think and the story you tell about your life. Your money and financial assets; your body's state of wellness, clarity, flexibility, size, and shape; your work environment, how you are treated, work satisfaction, and rewards—indeed, the very happiness of your life experience in general—is all happening because of the story that you tell."

Abraham

Who Would I Be without My Story?

When we change the emotional attachments we have to the pain, hurts and the betrayals of the past, then our identity changes.

But what if we are not willing to change our identity?

WHERE'S THE GRIEF?

I've had clients who were hesitant to lose their grief, suffering or resentments ... I suppose because those emotions had also become an integral part of their existence.

I recall one client who before our work together had an entire constellation of caretakers surrounding her, maintaining her status quo, keeping in place her identity of frailty: three medical doctors, a chiropractor, a massage therapist, and a reflexologist.

At her last session, she raised her major concern: how am I ever going to tell them I don't need them anymore?

WHO AM I NOW?

Another client was confused and upset that past recollections of past childhood abuses had faded to a point that *"I don't even know if they're real any more. Things are floating past. I can't get hold of my thoughts. They seem to be passing by outside of me, like a picture show, like I'm observing it as opposed to it being me."*

Her back pain had receded from 10 to zero on the intensity scale. That was the desired result. Yet she was upset at the loss of bad memories on which she had built her sense of self.

POOR, PITIFUL ME

People aren't always happy about the idea of giving up the "Poor Me" role and coming into their own power. In fact, there is often a great deal of resistance to it.

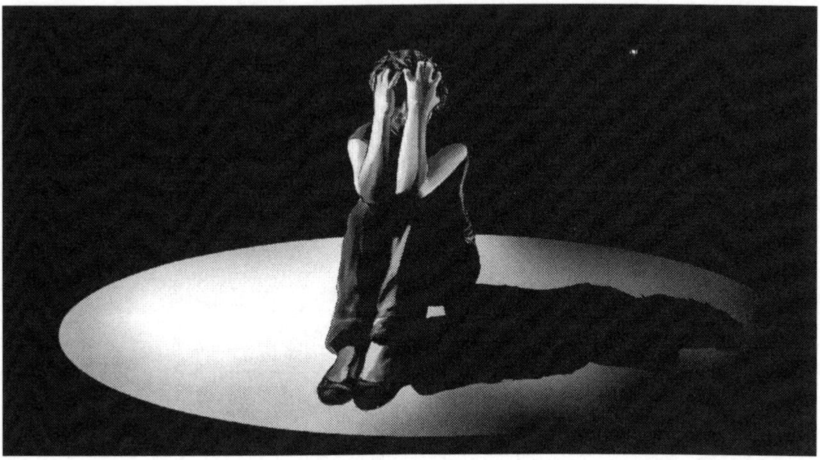

VICTIM

One client said to me, *"I'm very sad that I'm not a victim any more and I'm so upset with you for taking that away from me. F*** you."*

But all was forgiven, and in our next session, she was willing to work it through and change her identity from victim to powerhouse.

If you are so emotionally attached to your story that it has become part of the fabric of your identity, you are likely to encounter great resistance to detaching yourself.

You may initially find it a challenge even with the assistance of a practitioner.

IT'S A DECISION

At the risk of sounding simplistic, I think it's a matter of changing our mindset. It's making the decision to be strong, to design and take responsibility for our own life.

So if you want to reclaim your power, make that your goal. Set that intention.

Here are some suggested commands to your subconscious mind to use while tapping:

CLAIM YOUR POWER

Let go feeling sorry for myself.
Let go feeling like a victim.
Clear this feeling that life isn't fair.
I'm okay to let go of the victim role.
Let go blaming others for how I feel.
I'm the one doing this to me and I'm the one who's putting an end to it right now.
I gave away my power for most of my life.
Now I'm taking it back.
I built my life around it and now it's time for it to stop.
I forgive everyone.
Let go my story. I'm writing a new story.

Reason #23:

We Have Unrealistic Expectations

We tend to get impatient when tapping methods don't prove miraculous. But let's not forget that not too many years ago none of these methods was available to the lay population. You had to invest in costly and lengthy talk therapy that made you feel heard and understood but that often yielded dubious results.

That all changed in 1995 when Gary Craig made Emotional Freedom Techniques available to all, for a nominal fee.[3]

All the free YouTube videos posted by practitioners contribute to the new Internet mindset: I should be able to get it for free. Not only should I be able to get those same results for free and as easily and rapidly as I see on the videos, I should be able to accomplish this all on my own.

Transformation Takes Time

This is an unrealistic expectation because in the video the person is working with an objective, skilled facilitator who does not buy

3 Today, Gary Craig makes Optimal EFT™ available on the basis of voluntary donations: http://optimal-eft.emofree.com/. So generous.

into the person's story and who knows how to go in and make deep changes as fast as possible before the conscious mind can step in and gum up the works.

For one thing, only the spectacular sessions get posted. As I heard Gary Craig say in an interview, "People who don't get the dramatic results don't write about it."

Moreover, we're usually seeing only the final breakthrough portion of a session.

BELIEVING THAT EVERY SESSION RESULTS IN A MIRACLE CURE

A post by a colleague in a practitioner forum raised the question of the ethics of posting dramatic testimonials videotaped immediately after a group workshop where emotions were running high.

The fact that a person has had a major emotional shift doesn't mean that the person will never be triggered again. That too is an unrealistic expectation. One "tree" got rooted out. If there are more trees in the person's "forest" (and I can guarantee you there are if you suffer from childhood trauma or depression or addiction or any chronic illness) there's gonna be a lot more work to do.

As I wrote in Reason #13: There's never just one cockroach.

Believe in video testimonials that are taped days and weeks after the successful session.

Expecting the Same Results

It's always a mistake to compare ourselves to others and to think we can get those same results. Because we all hold memories and emotions in our own way. We all uniquely delete, distort and generalize our experiences. We all have our own triggers and patterns and perspectives.

This is true whether or not we're working with a practitioner.

Even a practitioner can't predict what your results will be. As a for instance, I treated a woman for childhood molestation. Within seven or eight months, she lost 80 lbs. Yet her weight had never entered the conversation.

Expecting Immediate Results Even with a Practitioner

Every practitioner loves to hear "You healed my life in one 2-hour session." I have my share of these. We all do and we love to quote them. But that's not a result we can expect with every client.

You don't necessarily get to a place of peace in one gulp when you have been depressed for 18 years or replaying your childhood trauma in memory several times a day. You will get there. You may need to be patient however.

Here's the thing …

We expect immediate results but it can take our neurological system time to absorb the deep changes. The brain needs time to reconfigure.

DON'T WORRY IF THE EARTH DOESN'T MOVE

Some of us make small, incremental changes. I confess I am one of them. In fact, I may just be a practitioner's worst nightmare because my progress seems to be more subdued and much less intense than most people's. This can be a bit unsettling for practitioners who work with me.

I was talking about this one day with a friend who is also a practitioner and she jokingly agreed with me about my failings as a client. She laughed, *"I wouldn't be calling you to illustrate a technique in front of a group. I'd be, like, 'Get out of that chair. Now! You're way too slow!'"*

So, while I have seen instant transformations happen with my own and other people's clients, it was not my path. The reason it took longer is that my core beliefs were entangled, hidden and deeply submerged. There were many, many protective layers to work through.

Some of us just take longer. That is why persistence is key.

DON'T BE TOO QUICK TO SAY YOU'RE NOT GETTING RESULTS

When "Dolores" contacted me she had already tried various modalities to rid herself of what she labeled "gut wrenching terror attacks," "panic" and "gut level fear" stemming from a dimly recalled childhood trauma. The first two-hour session was intense, as you can imagine.

As always, I had followed up in writing to ask how she was doing since our time together earlier in the month. Dolores' response was not as enthusiastic as I had anticipated. She said it had taken her three days to move through the experience. Her grieving and fears were not as long or as intense. She was still feeling depressed but was taking action to create meaningful work with her talents. (Interestingly, neither depression nor the issue of work had been mentioned in our session.)

The focus had shifted.

I wrote to her that our system can only handle so much in one 2-hour session. That is why it took her three days to move through the experience. I said that from my perspective she had made real progress since our first conversation. Her emotional state at the time was, in her words, "… for 4 – 5 hours a day tapping, grieving, crying, wailing, taking care of myself."

I told her I was very encouraged by what she had written. One layer gets taken care of and another emerges to be dealt with. There is always more work to be done to get to a place of peace.

This is just the latest example from my files. There is progress but it may not feel like progress for various reasons.

Tapping works. When it appears not to, we have to ask ourselves why.

1. Sometimes it's because of unrealistic expectations.
2. Or there's more work to be done.
3. Or the work we did made it safe for a deeper issue to emerge for clearing.

You are no doubt familiar with the onion metaphor—you first peel off the visible, superficial layer. It reveals another layer beneath. Another comes to the surface. You peel it off and another is revealed until you get to the heart.

4. Sometimes the changes in the brain (e.g. lessened anxiety, greater sense of personal freedom) happen so gently and rapidly and are so subtle that you do not realize or acknowledge that the issue has been resolved.

   So the person tends to forget or downplay or minimize the extent of distress he felt before our work together.

5. Sometimes the shift feels so natural that we are not aware of the change in ourselves that others notice.

I mentioned earlier that this is what Dr. Roger Callahan called The Apex Problem.

I call this …

"THE SUN IS SHINING SYNDROME"

One of my first EFT clients was my younger sister (the one my older sister and I apparently traumatized by dangling her upside down in a garbage can when she was little).

I worked with her to resolve some deep and long-standing issues that were threatening her marriage. These worries were causing her such anguish that she would constantly break into tears. The intensity of the emotion was affecting every aspect of her life.

There's more, but that's enough detail to set the scene.

After an intensive first session, she said, "Thank you. I feel lighter." And I noticed as she left the room that she walked just that much taller.

One week later, she came for her second session. The tension was gone from her face and she had a rosy skin tone. She looked happier than I had seen her in years.

Here's how the conversation went after she reported that nothing had changed:

Me: *You look 10 years younger than the last time I saw you.*

She: *Well, I feel good. It's spring. The sun is shining. And I took the dog for a walk in the park this morning.*

Me: *So, in the past three years that you have been suffering with this problem, not sleeping, crying all the time, was it ever spring? Did the sun ever shine? Did you ever take puppy for a walk in the park?* [I'm thinking ... would it kill you to give these methods a little credit here?]

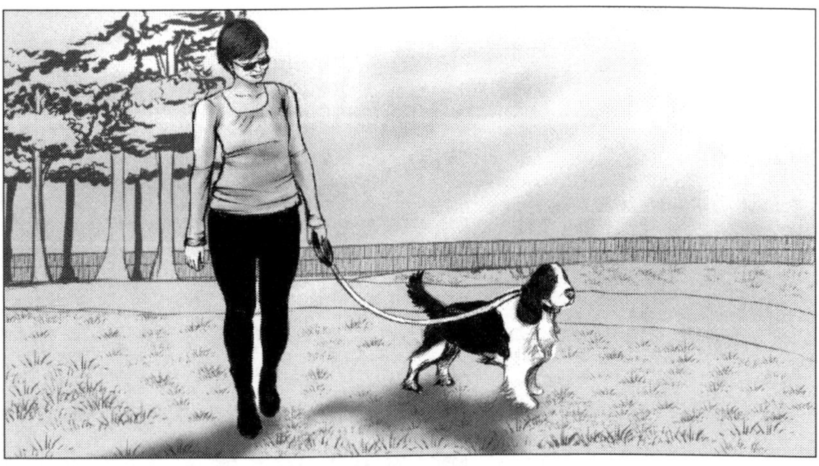

"WELL, I FEEL GOOD. IT'S SPRING. THE SUN IS SHINING. AND I TOOK THE DOG FOR A WALK IN THE PARK THIS MORNING."

She: [laughing and experiencing what we in the business call a "cognitive shift"] *Oh my gawd! That's too funny! I've been sleeping well. I haven't woken up crying even once.*

Me: *Yeah. Hilarious.* [I guess you can get away with sarcasm when the client is your younger sister!]

See why I call it "The Sun is Shining Syndrome?"

Needless to say, I am constantly having to set my ego aside and say, "This person's life is transformed. Get yourself (that would be *me*) out of the way!"

A shining sun is a wondrous thing. The mind healing itself in such a way that it feels normal is also a wondrous thing.

BONUS CHAPTER
BY ERIC B. ROBINS, M.D.

WHY TRANSFORMATION IS SUCH A CHALLENGE FROM A MEDICAL PERSPECTIVE

PEOPLE SAY THAT the body tends to heal itself, but my clinical experience shows that this might not always be the case. What I've come to learn in 25 years of incorporating mind-body healing techniques into a busy medical practice is that:

1. Early stressors and traumas can put our physiology into a fight-flight-freeze state, and can cause parts of our musculature to contract and spasm in order to protect us from becoming overwhelmed.

2. For many folks, this physiology then persists, almost going on autopilot, like a computer program continuously running underneath the surface. Then, every time in the future that there is a stressor or trigger, our brains and bodies react in this programmed "stressful" way.

3. Areas of our musculature can stay in a chronically tensed, armored state for months, years or decades, and in my opinion this is one of the biggest causes of energy blockage in the meridians and throughout the body.

4. According to Stanford cell biologist Dr. Bruce Lipton, when our systems are in a chronic stress state, the cells are in "survival" mode. It's only when we shift out of this chronic stress state that our cells can begin to "heal and regenerate."

5. Many emotional and mental problems seem to also arise from our physiology. I believe the science is starting to reflect a "bottoms up approach," meaning that when our physiology is in a chronic stress state, when our muscles and fasciae are chronically contracted, we feel bad, anxious, angry, depressed, fatigued, overwhelmed, etc.

6. The bottom line is this: If you want to heal from chronic emotional or physical illnesses or pain, then you have to shift your physiology out of a chronic stress state. The challenge is, to the best of my knowledge, there is nothing in standard allopathic medicine that does this.

7. An important key to shifting out of a chronic stress state is clearing the emotional charge off of past traumas, and working through the limiting core beliefs that filter our perceptions of life.

Sometimes Tapping Alone Isn't Enough

As word of my use of EFT in a medical setting spread, I began to get progressively more difficult cases referred to me. Some of these folks didn't seem to respond as well to basic tapping.

I began to look for ways to incorporate other principles and techniques into my sessions to make them faster and more effective.

What I found most useful were:

1. The understanding that the only thing that's real is now; if we have strong emotions or reactions coming up, and there is actually nothing happening at this moment to affect our safety and well-being, then we are in a hypnotic trance state (and experiencing conditioned neurological responses). And it's important to help our clients break free of this trance state (using tapping as well as other modalities such as TRE) in order that they can heal themselves.

2. When a client comes in with a problem, I'll ask them, "How do you know?" What I'm looking for ideally is having the client notice the raw physical sensations in their bodies, the presence of which tells them that there is a problem, that something is wrong.

   If they are able to do this (sometimes with coaching), then I ask them to allow the sensations to be there fully, to not attach meanings or labels to these sensations, to not judge them as good or bad, and to just tap on their awareness of the sensations. One mantra that I use, that makes it easier for folks to allow themselves to experience deeply painful emotions (without attributing blame, or finding reasons to not feel it) is, "It's okay to trust the truth of what you're feeling (as raw sensation), without attributing a why."

3. In NLP, we learn that for most problems, there is an underlying structure. How do folks internally go about having a problem? What is their underlying belief system that allows it to develop? What things are they doing in their neurology to make them feel so bad about X? Are they moving towards what they do want, or away from what they don't want? If they are moving away from what they don't

want, then they are holding this internal representation inside (and perhaps unknowingly adding emotional energy to it and attracting it). This can be identified and tapped on.

4. As quoted elsewhere in these pages, one of my hypnosis teachers, Stephen Parkhill once said, "No matter how much manure (trauma) you shovel out of the shed, in order for our clients to heal, we have to teach them to look for the good."

This lesson has been immensely useful for me personally as well as for my patients. One thing I've noticed is that most of my chronically ill patients are very good at feeling bad. They have deep "grooves" in their neural networks that allow them to easily notice what's not right, what still hurts, and how bad everything is in their lives.

The challenge is, when a person thinks thoughts like this, this mode of thinking puts them right back into stress mode again. And the increased levels of stress hormones sensitize pain fibers so that everything hurts more. Also, stress hormones increase inflammation in the body and affect the normal function of our immune system.

Therefore, it is incumbent on us to not just tap away at trauma, but also to inspire and mentor our clients to begin to notice what's good in their lives. This can take time and can actually feel very foreign to many people.

Another Parkhill quote that helps elucidate this, "Security is not what feels good, it's what feels familiar." We have to assist our clients in becoming comfortable with new ways of thinking and feeling and being.

I recommend that folks spend 5-10 minutes per day thinking about what they appreciate and are grateful for. With many folks, this is exceedingly difficult and yet we must help them and teach them to develop this part of their neurology—the feeling good part. Some of my patients in the beginning were able to notice that only their little toe on their left foot felt comfortable and free and safe in this moment. If this is the case, then we shift their attention to how good the little toe feels. It's a process and we build from there.

Renowned EFT teacher Silvia Hartmann also realizes that complete healing is not always just about clearing away trauma, and has based her Positive EFT system on this. Positive EFT is a combination of having folks begin to generate and focus on positive feelings, and then using tapping to both anchor those positive feeling states and also to increase energy flow through the body. I'm so delighted that Mia has a section on Positive EFT in this book, and understands these important principles as well.

Eric B. Robins, M.D.
Urologist and Mind-Body Healing Specialist
Co-author, "Your Hands Can Heal You"

PART II:

QUESTIONS AND ANSWERS

WHO GETS RESULTS ON THEIR OWN?

WHY DO I SOMETIMES FEEL WORSE WHEN TAPPING?

WHY DO YOU FEEL THAT WORDS ARE NOT IMPORTANT WHEN TAPPING?

HOW DO I KNOW THE TAPPING WAS SUCCESSFUL?

WHEN SHOULD I THINK OF WORKING WITH A TAPPING PRACTITIONER RATHER THAN FLYING SOLO?

WHY IS IT SO DIFFICULT TO DO ON MY OWN?

WHY DO PEOPLE AROUND US CHANGE WHEN WE DO?

WHAT IF I NEED A PRACTITIONER AND AM UNABLE TO PAY?

Q: Who Gets Results on Their Own?

A: In my experience, it's a tiny percentage of people who can get deep results working on their own. Five percent, maybe? Another 15-20 percent of people can get 80 percent results on their own or in just a session or two with a good practitioner.

It's a very general statement, I know, but that is the conclusion I've come to after several years in the field.

The purpose of this book, and Part III in specific, is to show you, step by step, how to get the most out of your tapping efforts.

Q: Who Are the 20%?

A: Those who get results on their own are the people whose issues are not as deep-seated as yours. They are the select few who have little internal resistance to positive change. Little resistance to letting go of negative memories from the past. Little resistance to reimprinting the bad with good jiu-jitsu.

Once they resolve and replace their worst negative life experiences with new positive references the rest falls away and takes care of itself in a sort of ripple effect. Life is good.

Who are these fortunate people?

People who came from a stable, fairly happy home, who felt treasured as infants, who knew their parents loved them and did the best they knew how. They have fewer bad memories and negative emotions to begin with. They had a rather easy life until some trauma or other erupted and threw their life in turmoil.

I wish I were one of them.

Don't you?

Q: HOW ABOUT THE OTHER 80%?

A: The other 80 percent get only 20 percent results on their own. They may get results at the start. Then the results stop. Most often, it's because once the surface level gets dealt with, they hit a wall of fear and the old survival mechanism kicks in. So they are unable to get to the core issues without professional help.

Or they get results and feel so much better than before that they quit too soon and never fully experience the true benefit of these methods.

Or they discover that it isn't roses all the way because as old patterns begin to crumble and dissolve, underlying emotions and beliefs are now free to bubble to the surface to be cleared.

There's simply more work to do.

Some may conclude that meridian tapping doesn't work and feel like giving up. Others persist in spite of poor results, encouraged by the stunning results they see in others.

The smart ones seek assistance from a qualified practitioner because it's almost impossible for most of us to get beyond the 20% without a trusted, experienced guide.

HEART CONNECTION

There is something to be said for connecting with an experienced practitioner, in a bond of trust, feeling understood and allowing the person to guide us down paths that, working on our own, we unconsciously avoid.

In my own personal experience with tapping, something happens when I'm working with someone else that does not happen when I'm working on my own. It's like a third presence.

Very often, it's the heart connection which develops between client and practitioner that contributes to the healing process.

Q: WHY DO I SOMETIMES FEEL WORSE WHEN TAPPING?

A: You may temporarily feel worse when you have tapped into (excuse the pun) a deep issue that takes a bit longer to resolve.

One of my current clients reports that she feels like she's been hit by a truck after our sessions. She also mysteriously develops swelling of the right side of her face almost every time we work together.

It's a sign that the tapping is working at a profound level.

From my experience, if when tapping you feel worse than before, you probably need the guidance of a practitioner.

Tapping will always make you feel better … eventually. And that's where persistence pays off.

Q: WHY DO YOU FEEL THAT WORDS ARE NOT IMPORTANT WHEN TAPPING?

A: While there is energy attached to words (everything is energy, as you know), words can keep you in your head and make you overthink things.

In Reason #23, I referred to the onion metaphor. You peel off layers until you get to the heart. Often at the heart are issues that reflect back to infancy and the pre-verbal stages of childhood.

Beyond that, you might think of the onion as an energetic structure. Many people believe that these energetic layers originated over several generations. If we're born with inherited beliefs and imprints, words are likely not too effective in changing them.

Tapping works best when we focus on the body sensations, the gut reactions. You don't want to let words get in the way. Worrying about what words to use will only obstruct your progress.

Q: HOW DO I KNOW THE TAPPING WAS SUCCESSFUL?

I'll answer this question with one last story …

The week I was writing these final chapters I had a first session with a man in his late 20's who described himself as *"susceptible to a cycle of self-deprecation and self-destruction."*

We worked through four unresolved traumatic episodes from his early years. One episode involved harsh discipline and shaming by his kindergarten teacher who wanted to teach him a lesson for consistently leaving his gym clothes at home.

"Jack" was a rebellious little kid who was *"constantly at odds with every teacher I can remember."*

He said, *"I was stripped to my underwear in front of the class during gym."*

We worked through the child's feelings of humiliation, shame, panic, sadness, unfairness, lack of protection and other associated emotions, including the sense he could never trust anyone.

When we were at zero, I asked him how he would have this story end if he had had control of the situation. He saw himself in the gym, happily practicing shooting basketballs into the net.

He said, *"What I appreciate about today is creating visualizations where I can trust in myself and come to my own rescue in those instances where I didn't have control. I can retroactively take control."*

I asked Jack whether I might include his story in a book I was writing. He declined, saying the whole thing was too humiliating.

The next morning I received this message in my inbox:

> *I'd like you to go ahead and use that story in your book if you like, I changed my mind. It's funny because it no longer really embarrasses me, I don't mind. I think it'd be funny to read it someday! Since I will only remember shooting hoops with myself anyway.*

A: You know the tapping was successful when …

1. You feel you are now in control of the situation.

2. You still have the memory but there's no emotion attached to it. The negativity is gone. All emotional triggers have evaporated. The feeling is one of neutrality and detachment (and sometimes, humor).

3. It doesn't resonate any more when you replay the scene in your mind days, weeks and months later. *That is the true test.*

Do keep in mind, however, that you have cleared one specific episode. If you're like most people, there is more work to be done to get to a happy place.

Q: When Should I Think of Working with a Tapping Practitioner Rather Than Flying Solo?

A: You know you need private sessions when …

- You are feeling dissociated and are not getting ahead in spite of regularly tapping on your own.

- You are a victim of rape, sexual violence or molestation, including early introduction to sexuality.

- You were consistently given messages in your family that you didn't matter: "Why would anybody like you?" "You're so stupid." "It's no wonder you're always the last one picked for a team." You are unable to shake the memory of an attack or a trauma such as a deadly motor vehicle accident.

- You are unable to move through the unbearable pain of the death of a child.

- You have never healed from the death of one or both of your parents at an early age.
- You can't recognize your hidden psychological triggers.
- You suffer from what one of my clients called "a crippling anxiety."
- You have had or feel you are about to have a nervous breakdown.
- You suffer from PTSD (Post-Traumatic Stress Disorder).
- You suffer from FM (Fibromyalgia), MS (Multiple Sclerosis), ME/CFS (Myalgic Encephalomyelitis/Chronic Fatigue Syndrome), MCS (Multiple Chemical Sensitivity), EI (Environmental Illness) or another "hidden disability" or autoimmune disease.

Don't let video testimonials recorded immediately after a one or two-hour session deceive you into believing in a miracle cure. Chronic diseases and addictions have very deep roots and require extensive treatment.

- You were abused or bullied in childhood.[x]
- You have self-destructive tendencies or behaviors. Like a client of mine who was literally pulling out her hair due to job stress, another who found cutting less painful than confronting the ache inside, and yet another who was toying with thoughts of ending her life.
- You are so emotionally exhausted that you are running on fumes.

- You are resistant to tapping. (This often takes the form of "forgetting" to tap.)

- Your anxiety is all-pervasive and permeates every aspect of your life.

- You say you don't have visual memory. I can tell you from personal experience, because that was the case with me, that lack of visual memory is a sign of big fear. (However, memories can be accessed through other senses, as I discuss in Reason #3: Because we're unable to get to the structure of the problem on our own.)

- You have been trying to lose weight for years and have tried everything, without being able to control your cravings.

- You cannot remember a time when you felt deeply loved and cherished.

- You were psychologically mistreated, or feel you were neglected or emotionally abandoned when you were young. Deep emotional scars on the psyche of a small child cause a feeling of not being safe in the world.

- You have spent a lifetime suppressing your early emotions.

- You have an over-developed sense of responsibility for everything and everyone around you.

- You're engaged in what one of my clients named a "deadly little dance."

All the above reasons that I feel you should work privately with a practitioner are based on my personal client files. And my own personal journey.

Again, other practitioners will have had experiences different to mine and may disagree with me.

Q: Why Is It so Difficult to Do on My Own?

A: There is only so much we can do, working on ourselves. Sometimes we are afraid to go into uncharted areas all alone. We lose our way. We avoid delving as deep as we need to in order to make deep changes.

"Deadly Little Dance"

I recently worked with "Sherry" who had been tapping daily for two years on her own. She could pinpoint all her repetitive life themes, which included "loser" and "I'm all alone."

She had been tapping on emotions which included anger, shame, guilt, betrayal, worthlessness, low self-esteem, neglect, and rejection. Without success.

When Sherry contacted me it was at a moment of crisis in her life. After our session, she told me in rather poetic terms that her issues had all been "*caught up in a swirl in a deadly little dance.*" She said, "I'm very surprised at the pain issues we addressed."

Are your issues all caught up in a swirl in a deadly little dance? If so, it may be near impossible to get to the heart of it on your own.

ON THE OTHER HAND …

If you and a practitioner dislodge something big you may more easily work through remaining fragments on your own.

DON'T FEEL BAD IF YOU AREN'T ABLE TO DO IT ON YOUR OWN

Even we practitioners will often seek assistance because what we can do for other people we are unable to do for ourselves. That certainly was true in my case.

My clients always express surprise when I tell them that I needed to work with an objective, trusted third party to get to the source of my own misery.

On one of the EFT forums I subscribe to, a fellow practitioner wrote:

> … *I am in great need of recovery from CFS* [Chronic Fatigue Syndrome]. *I'm a very accomplished EFT Practitioner, but as we all know, working with yourself can be challenging-to-ineffective on the big stuff.*

That could be my story. I'd love to be able to say that I got to a happy place in just a few sessions or that that I was able to do it on my own. But that would not be true. For me, it was a journey, and by no means an instant transformation.

I *have* been able to clear up fragments of issues on my own with meridian tapping. But not all. I've needed help with the larger issues such as overcoming early childhood violence, rape, betrayals and lingering financial losses, to name just a few.

If even seasoned practitioners find it a challenge to work on themselves, how much more difficult for the layperson?

No problem can be solved from the same level of consciousness that created it.

ALBERT EINSTEIN, 1879-1955

Q: Why Do People Around Us Change When We Do?

You stated that one of the virtues of doing this work is that when we change at a deep, fundamental level, the people around us change and everything in our universe begins to transform. What is the explanation of why this happens?

A: We live in a holographic universe. The brain is part of the hologram. "All things in the universe are infinitely interconnected."[xi]

That is why when we make a positive change, the world around us reflects that positive change. It's a miraculous thing.

Q: What If I Need a Practitioner and Am Unable to Pay?

New practitioners who require a certain number of hours to qualify for the various certification levels may be happy to work with you at reduced rates. Get yourself accepted into one of the open groups on Facebook and post a notice asking for this sort of assistance.

This is Important

On the topic of working with a third party, just make sure that the person you select to work with doesn't have your issues. Because if the practitioner has the same issues and identifies with you, your issues will not go away. They may only be reinforced.

And now, you're asking, how would I know if the person has my issues? Ask the person whether they have had your issue or anything like it and how they feel about it now. If you sense any heaviness or negative emotion at all. If the language suggests anything other than "it happened," "I'm done with it" or "it's all good" then you know the problem has not been fully dealt with. And keep looking.

PART III:

Unlocking the Secrets to Your Tapping Success

For Best Results Working on Your Own

Meridian Tapping Points

How to Tap

9-Step Process to Clear the Structure of a Problem

Give Context to Negative Emotions

NLP and Working with Your Memories

Unscientific, Untested Approach to Deleting Negative Fractals

Tap on Your Child Self

Questions to Ask Yourself if You Get Stuck

When You Don't Know What to Say While Tapping

Ask & Receive

Focus on the Good

Positive EFT

Positive EFT as a Meditation

For Best Results Working on Your Own

1. Hydration is important. Always drink water when you are doing this work.

2. For best results, focus on specific events and their details.

3. Make every effort to treat the belief, memory or situation as not real. It is helpful to remind yourself that (1) the event happened in the past, (2) it has no power over you because you realize it's not happening in this present moment, and (3) you're safe in this present moment. This is important because safety is a huge issue.

4. Write down a number between 1 and 10 that represents the intensity of the emotion as you remember the event. Mentally put yourself back into the negative situation. Bring the memory into full consciousness and note where it lodges in your body.

5. Go at it with what Gary Craig calls "surgical precision":

   Break every event into its various components. EFT calls them "aspects." Deal with every detail, however insignificant it may seem. Every facet of the memory. Every twist and turn. Every facial expression. Every sound, taste, smell. If it comes up now, it was significant at the time and needs to be cleared.

6. Allow yourself to feel the emotions that arise, and tap them down to zero.

   Make sure you resolve to zero every bit that comes up. Otherwise the issue will resurface in another way.

7. Treat any image or memory or emotion or metaphor that pops in as attached to the issue you're working on.

8. The key is connecting to an intense emotion as you tap in order to create change at a deep, unconscious, cellular level.

   It's too easy to lapse into naming emotions in an effort to cover all bases, rather than allowing ourselves to feel them in order to uproot and evaporate them.

9. Be persistent. Sometimes you just have to go at it like a terrier with a bone.

10. Test: "Am I at zero?" Go back into the experience in great detail. Don't worry that you will undermine the work you have done because done properly, the pieces you successfully resolved will not recur. If a thing appears to recur, it only means there's more to do.

    Deal with any new, related issues that come to the surface to be treated.

11. Then you have to test again. Test the next day, the next week, the next month.

Chances are the whole issue will have dissolved into insignificance. When that happens, you know you have succeeded.

12. Sometimes the shifts feel so natural we're not aware of changes that have taken place. It's easy to conclude that you haven't made the changes you were hoping for. I dealt with this topic in Part I: Reason #23: We have unrealistic expectations.

    So keep a record or journal of your ongoing progress. Start by recording how you feel *before* your tapping sessions and after.

Meridian Tapping Points

As you know, we tap on easily accessible end points of meridians.

The usual tapping points include side of hand, inner eyebrow, outer eye, under eye, under nose, under mouth, and under armpit. Many add the "one hundred meeting point" at the top of the head. Some practitioners include the liver point (under the breast).

Others include the gamut point (between and beneath the knuckles of the ring and little fingers) as part of the 9 Gamut Procedure.

SET (Simple Energy Techniques) includes tapping on finger points at the base of the nail, on the thumb side, as well as the side of the hand to help absorb the shocks of everyday life. The idea is to use a lot of continual meridian stimulation as a form of "general energy toning." [xii]

Many of us prefer to keep it simple with just 5 points: forehead, outer eye, under eye, under collarbone, and wrist.

We practitioners seem to all have our preferences. But the secret to tapping success is not which points you use. If you experiment with this you will see that you get results if you tap almost anywhere. Just keep it simple and tap on various points as you focus on feelings and body sensations.

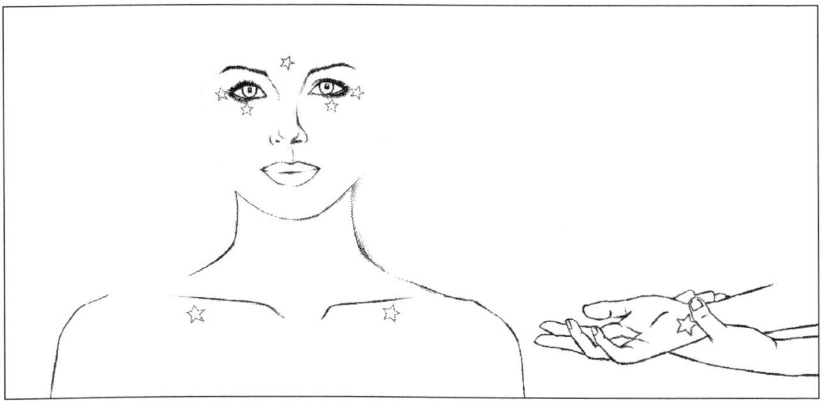

5 TAPPING POINTS

And here is where I may annoy a lot of EFT practitioners who have been trained on the value of tapping on the "KC" point (side of the hand) while making three setup statements that start with "Even though."

While you could argue that this work requires empathy and the framing statement "Even though … I deeply and completely love and accept myself" reflects compassion for self and acceptance of the inner conflict that causes us to act in ways that contradict a desired state, I don't believe it is necessary to endlessly repeat the words in order to feel compassion and acceptance of oneself. Your subconscious knows your intention.

In my opinion, this is an outdated, cumbersome ritual that adds nothing to an otherwise elegant method. If you can get the same excellent results without the ritual, why add complexity?

> *In every culture and in every medical tradition before ours, healing was accomplished by moving energy.*
>
> ALBERT SZENT-GYÖRGYI, WINNER OF NOBEL PRIZE IN PHYSIOLOGY OR MEDICINE (1893 – 1986)

How to Tap

Practitioners all have their preferences. But really, you can tap with one, two, three or four fingertips of one hand or both hands. You can tap on the right or left side of the body or crosswise. It doesn't matter. The sequence in which you tap doesn't matter.

You can tap or rub or press and hold the acupressure points. It's the act of stimulating the points that produces the magic of releasing negative emotions, lowering anxiety and harmful cortisol levels, boosting the immune system, increasing cell repair hormones, lowering blood pressure, and rewiring our brain.

The amount of pressure you use isn't important. In fact, once your body is familiar with the tapping sensation, I have found that even imagining yourself tapping works for most people.

It isn't the words you use, either. And it isn't a matter of repeating positive statements. It's a matter of focusing on a belief or thought or feeling or problem and where it registers in the body.

Compassion for ourselves while tapping is crucial.

Noticing what is going on in our body and tapping on those physical sensations is also key. Tap wherever it takes you.

Tap any time you want to shake off a negative feeling and keep it from taking hold. Tap until you feel lighter and freer.

9-STEP PROCESS TO CLEAR THE STRUCTURE OF A PROBLEM

NOTE: As mentioned earlier, I do not suggest that you work alone on traumatic and deeply upsetting life episodes because of the danger of retriggering the suffering. Work with a skilled practitioner.

1. Start by setting a specific goal or intention for this session with yourself. What specific problem (heartbreak, shame, anxiety … whatever) do you want to clear, once and for all?

2. Select one specific event or memory to process. [See Part III: Give context to negative emotions.]

3. As you recall the memory, assign a number representing the intensity of your emotion on a scale of 1 (low) – 10 (high).

4. Ask, "How does it make me feel? *Where* do I feel it in my body?"

   You are not looking for the *cause* of the problem, only your *feeling response* to it.

5. Start at the beginning and replay the memory, focusing on the details of what you saw and heard and felt.

Go at it piece by piece, tapping on the meridian points.

Don't be concerned whether the details are accurate or not. It doesn't matter because it's how you represent the experience in your mind.

You are tapping to disconnect the *emotion* you feel as you recall the memory. You do not need to name the emotion.

Don't worry about the words. You don't need a script. You just need to allow yourself to *feel* it.

6. Tap on your body's *physical response* to the memory *(tightness in my chest | pounding in my ears | lump in my throat).* You can just say, *"Whatever this is, whatever the cause, whatever the source, whatever it represents, I give myself permission to let it go."* Or *"Clear it!"* Tap until it feels better.

7. Hold your wrist, with thumb on the pulse points. Take a long, slow, deep breath in. Exhale slowly and gently.

8. Go back to the memory and check the level of intensity on the 1 – 10 scale. The reason for doing this is to assess your progress. Tap on what is left until you get to zero or close to it. (*Clear all remaining tightness in my chest. | Let go of everything that supports this memory.)*

Your goal is to tap every aspect of the memory down to zero. You will know you have succeeded when you replay the memory and it has no emotional trigger. It doesn't resonate any more. Where it used to distress you it now means nothing to you. The negativity is completely gone. You feel indifferent to it.

9. Once that is done, the last important step is to go back inside the memory and replace it with a happy one. In a perfect world, how would you have the story end?

   That's the new memory you want to install. If you don't have a happy memory to draw from, make one up.

   (This works because, as you have no doubt read, the mind/body does not know the difference between imagination and reality.) The response is the same.

   The true test is that hours, days, weeks, months and years hence you feel disconnected from the problem.

   One of the truly wondrous traits of this work is that, when you have cleared the negative structure of a problem, the positive changes are permanent.

GIVE CONTEXT TO NEGATIVE EMOTIONS

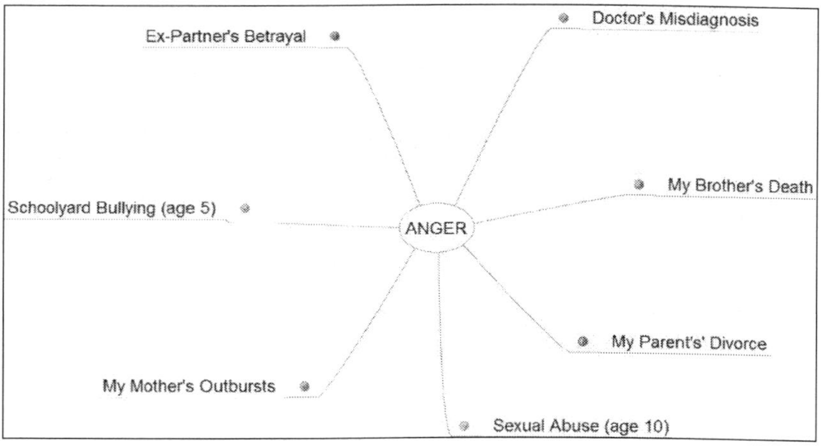

NEGATIVE EMOTION VISUAL CHART

1. Make a visual chart. In the center of the page, name the negative emotion you want to be rid of: anger/resentment/jealousy/guilt/ loss/abandonment/ sadness/rejection/shame ... or any other).

2. Draw spokes out from the center. Along each spoke, write a few words to identify a memory that supports that emotion.

3. Treat each memory or episode separately, following the protocol outlined in the 9-Step Process to Clear the Structure of a Problem (Part III).

4. Start with one memory. Tap to zero *every* aspect of the memory.

5. Other emotions will pop up.[4] Deal with every body sensation that surfaces and keep coming back to the emotion at the center of the chart.

6. Replay the episode from beginning to end, tapping on anything that remains until you feel no emotional charge.

7. Look back on the memory days later. You know you've done a great job if you can say something like, "*It happened. I'm done with it.*" Or "*It doesn't resonate any more.*"

   Transformation takes time. While sometimes change is instantaneous, more often healing happens in layers. So do not expect a quick fix.

4 Expect anything and follow where the emotions take you. The week I was writing this chapter I worked with a woman who had deep anger toward her mother. It was a 10 on the intensity scale. She reported that the sensation of anger lodged in her heart. For over an hour we focused only on the physical sensations. The sensations shifted from anger to sadness to "heavy sadness" to grief to abandonment to feeling blocked to burning "like a rug burn" in her throat to (strangely) a visible puffiness on the right side of her face to all the above emotions "popping in and out in little spurts" to an ache to a feeling of total exhaustion.

At the end of our appointment, when I asked about the anger and each of the above feelings in turn, she responded "Right now the anger doesn't exist. It's gone."

I strongly suggested she have a tall glass of water and allow herself to rest.

At our next session she told me that, while she never sleeps during the day, she was so exhausted after our session that she had needed two naps that afternoon.

NLP and Working with Your Memories

The founders of NLP (Neuro-Linguistic Programming) discovered that there are set ways that our brains encode and represent in memory the things that happen to us. These set ways of mentally processing information also govern how we learn and how we communicate.

For our purposes here – freeing ourselves of bad memories – we are concerned only with the things we do inside our head when recalling events from the past.

It all has to do with how the mind recorded, replays and gives meaning to those events.

Working within the systems in which we internally represent and reproduce our memories is the easiest way to affect change.

Representational Systems

The Representational Systems are usually referred to as VAK (Visual/Auditory/ Kinaesthetic). If we include Olfactory (smell) and Gustatory (taste) they are referred to as VAKOG.

There is another less common and less recognized modality called Auditory Digital (AD).

I am very familiar with this representational system because for decades I have worked with engineers, corporate and business people.

In my opinion, this is the most challenging of the systems for most practitioners to work with because we have to get people out of their heads and into the sights and sounds and feelings of a memory. It's not so easy for the AD to express deep emotion. (One of my clients described herself as "an emotional compactor." That about describes it!)

The following suggestions for working with your preferred representational system are to be used in tandem with the 9-Step Process to Clear the Structure of a Problem.

Are You Visual?

Do you see pictures in your mind's eye? Then you are very fortunate because the mind thinks in pictures.

You have a lot to work with: As you bring a memory to mind, do you see it in color or in black and white? Is it near or far away? Is the picture clear or fuzzy? Is it close up or panoramic? Sharply focused or out of focus? Bright or faded? Is it a still frame such as a photo or drawing? Is it 3 dimensional or flat?

Are you inside the picture or are you a spectator (looking in from outside the frame)? Or do you see it like a movie? Are you in the movie or are you watching as an observer? Who else is in the picture?

What you want to do is play with the picture. If in black and white, switch it to color. If it's far away, bring it close. If you see yourself as a spectator step into the picture. You want to be in it completely.

If it's a movie, you can run it backwards.

Look at the expressions on your own and other people's faces. Tap until the expressions change to positive and everybody is happy.

AUDITORY

Do you talk to yourself? Is there constant dialogue rattling around in your head? Do thoughts whisper in your ears? Do you replay earlier or imaginary conversations in your head, like I do?

What story do you tell yourself about the memory?

Do you hear someone else's words or your own words? Is it your voice or someone else's?

What are the words? What is the tone of voice? Is the voice loud or soft? What is the voice inflection?

Where is the sound coming from? Are there other sounds in the background?

A fun thing you can do to rid yourself of painful things that were said is to give a cartoon voice to each character in the memory. As corny as this sounds, it works because it breaks the negative association.

KINAESTHETIC

When you replay the memory in your mind, what do you *feel*? Where in your body do you feel the sensation? Is there a specific location? Is it an ache? A pain? A sharp pain? Throbbing? Is it pressure?

Are you aware of any textures or temperature changes?

Can you associate an emotion with it? Aim your tapping at the *physical sensation* of the emotion. (For example, aim at dissolving the burning rage at the back of your throat.)

AUDITORY DIGITAL

Rather than re-experiencing a memory, do you turn the information you received through your senses into language? Like the Auditory, do you mentally debate and carry on conversations with yourself and others in your head?

Do you like working with logical facts, analyzing, organizing, categorizing, summarizing, and figuring things out? Do you learn, not through mental pictures or your other five senses but via flow charts, nuts and bolts methods, procedures, logistics, systems, steps and sequences? Are you the sort of person who needs to understand and to think things through before commenting or making a decision?

If you are Auditory Digital, you will need to keep reminding yourself to turn off the internal dialogue and to tap on the *feelings* that the memory evokes. You will get results only if you can get to the buried emotion.

Unscientific, Untested Approach to Deleting Negative Fractals

1. Direct your subconscious mind: "My intention is to delete this pattern of "X."

2. Identify the symptoms of the negative pattern you want to delete. (Make a written list of all the ways the negative pattern manifests in your life. Or use the approach outlined in Give Context To Negative Emotions, Part III.)

3. In your mind's eye, see your negative pattern as a fractal. What you want to do here is make the invisible visible. Observe it without judging. If, like me, you are not a person who visualizes easily, have an image of a fractal in front of you. A simple Google search will yield hundreds to choose from.[xiii]

4. Allow yourself to *feel* the raw emotion (the anger, rage, fear, sadness) that is a *symptom* of the negative pattern. Accessing the raw emotion is the most important part of this process.

5. Tap on the meridian points as you focus on the *raw emotion*.

6. If you feel you need some words to direct your tapping:

- *I command my subconscious mind to release this imprint.*
- *Dissolve the pattern at its deepest roots.*
- *Clear the core root.*
- *Clear the cause of this problem.*
- *Let it go at source.*

7. See the pattern breaking up as you tap and dissolving at its deepest roots.

8. When the pattern has disappeared, see yourself reconstructing an opposite *positive* fractal. This is important.

9. Instruct your subconscious mind to accept the new pattern and to run the new pattern as a continuous positive loop.

Tap on Your Child Self

1. Go into your story and make a list of painful episodes from your childhood. Or make a visual chart, drawing spokes out from the center, as outlined earlier in Part III: Give context to negative emotions.

2. Treat each instance separately.

3. What did you as a child *feel* at the time?

4. Tap to zero all the feelings that come up, allowing the child to fully vent his emotions.

   Zoom out. Tap with objective compassion from the perspective of the adult who knows that it's all in the past. The child didn't feel safe then. But this is now. The child survived and is now safe. You are there to reassure and keep him safe:

   - *You are safe.*
   - *It's safe to let it go.*
   - *You're allowed to let it go.*

5. When you have tapped to zero, step into the picture as your adult self, there to love, guide and protect the child to a happier future.

6. Tell the child a secret, something that will empower him for the rest of his life. Tell him something you wish he had known all those years ago, that he can now carry over into his future.

7. Test your results. If there is any emotional residue, tap it away.

Questions to Ask Yourself if You Get Stuck

- *Why can't I let this go?*
- *What is the resistance to letting this go?*
- *I must be getting something out of it. What is it?*
- *What would happen if I were to let go of this problem?*
- *What is it about this that it doesn't feel safe?*
- *What does (this emotion) remind me of?*
- *If I were to be really honest with myself, what benefit do I get by having this problem?*
- *What am I avoiding by having this problem?*
- *If the problem went away, what is the worst thing that could happen to me?*
- *Would I know who I am if I didn't have this problem?*
- *Why is it important not to have this problem?*
- *If I were not emotionally connected to this situation, is there any chance I might view it differently?*
- *If I were to look at this objectively, in a way that didn't involve me personally, is there anything about this situation that is even in the least bit funny?*

See also: Part III: When you don't know what to say while tapping

When You Don't Know What to Say While Tapping

While I don't believe in the value of generic scripts, it's very useful to have a few key phrases to fall back on while tapping.

Following are direct commands to the subconscious mind that you might find useful when you are dealing with resistance, safety issues, trauma and difficulty forgiving.

THIS IS KEY: It's important to not get lost in the words. Allow yourself to *feel* the impact of the words in your body.

Resistance

[Note that in dealing with resistance, we want to accept the resistance as normal and natural, since the subconscious is trying to protect us. We acknowledge that its purpose is to keep us safe. Then we detach and release to melt it away.]

- *This is just resistance ...*
- *It wants to keep me safe ...*
- *I accept that there is a part of me that does not feel safe clearing this issue ...*
- *I accept that I am unwilling to change at this time ...*
- *I am fine exactly as I am ...*

Resistance (continued)

- *I am safe …*
- *I'm here in the present and I'm safe …*
- *I am safe to release …*
- *It's safe to let it go …*
- *I'm safe to let it go …*
- *It's safe to let go of the past …*
- *It's safe to let go all that it represents …*
- *Delete all attachment to this episode …*
- *I forgive myself for hanging on …*
- *Let go the habit of resistance …*
- *Whatever the fear behind the resistance …*
- *I'm allowed to let this go …*
- *I give myself permission to lovingly release it …*
- *I am choosing to release it …*
- *This is my choice. This is my command.*

Trauma[5]

- *I am safe to release this trauma …*
- *Let go the belief that I need to hold on to this trauma …*
- *Let go the impact of this experience on my body …*
- *Let go the shock of this trauma …*
- *Let go the shock at a cellular level …*
- *I let go the need to suffer …*
- *I let go the belief that I need to suffer …*
- *I release and let it go …*

Forgiveness

As writer Anne Lamott famously said, "*Not forgiving is like drinking rat poison and then waiting for the rat to die.*"

---

5 Again, I would not suggest that anyone attempt to tap on traumatic memories of war atrocities, natural disasters, terrorist events, mass violence or serious accidents on their own.

Forgiving is just releasing. Think of it as releasing the need to drink a poison that hurts only you.

It does not imply that we condone other people's bad behavior. It doesn't mean we haven't suffered as a result of what a person said, or did, or didn't do. It just means refusing to allow a person who has hurt you to still have power over you.

Coming to this realization was a turning point in my life. My hope is that it will do the same for you:

- *I forgive myself for hanging on ...*
- *I forgive everything connected to this memory ...*
- *I forgive [each individual person, dead or alive, who had anything to do with the episode ...*
- *Let go the need to hang on ...*
- *Release all judgment ...*
- *Delete all attachment to this episode ...*
- *Let go feeling like a victim ...*

Getting to the Root Cause

- *Clear this (name the problem) ...*
- *Whatever the underlying reason, heal it.*
- *Whatever the underlying tendency*
- *Whatever the underlying cause*
- *Whatever the underlying foundation ...*
- *If this is just a symptom of something deeper, clear it ...*
- *Whatever that is ...*
- *Whatever the imbalance ...*
- *Whatever the life theme ...*
- *Clear the imprint ...*
- *Clear the core root ...*

Ask & Receive

Ask and Receive is based on the idea that higher states of our consciousness always have the answers. It gently gives us access to this knowledge and facilitates change at a deep level.

1. Identify a limiting belief that is causing issues in your life and that you would like to eliminate.

   (a) As you think of it, rate the intensity of your emotion on a scale of 0 – 10.

   (b) Write the exact words you say to yourself when you think of it. These are the words [the limiting belief] you will use in the following tapping rounds.

   (c) From the heart, rate how true the sentence feels to you right now. A rating of 10 means it's absolutely true.

2. Tapping: Round 1

   There is a part of my being that already knows that I no longer need to believe [the limiting belief]. That part of my being is willing to inform the rest of me now. It is doing so now with grace and ease. My mind, body and spirit are receiving the information. Information transfer is now complete.

3. Test

State the limiting belief again, in the exact words you wrote. How does it feel now? Does it still feel as intense as the number you assigned? Has anything changed?

4. Tapping: Round 2

Even though this was true for me at the time, I no longer need to believe [the limiting belief]. And the part of my being that knows that is willing to inform the rest of me now. It is doing so now with grace and ease. My mind, body and spirit are receiving the information. Information transfer is now complete.

5. Test Again

6. Tapping: Round 3

There is a part of my being that already knows that it is perfectly safe for me to let go that old belief. And the part of my being that knows that is willing to inform the rest of me now. It is doing so now with grace and ease. My mind, body and spirit are receiving the information. Information transfer is now complete.

7. End Goal

You want the limiting belief at zero and the belief that you are perfectly safe to let it go to ring 100% true.

Focus on the Good

If you want to fully resolve an emotional issue, tapping is a good place to start. If you want to transform your world, you want to keep your focus on the good in your life.

Do this and the results will amaze you:

1. First thing in the morning, set the intention to have a happy day.
2. Repeat the old and famous optimistic autosuggestion of Émil Coué (1857 –1926), "Every day in every way, I am getting better and better." Say it often and as though you believe it.
3. Any time during the day, think of one thing you're deeply grateful for and hold the feeling for as long as you can.
4. Before bed, reflect on things that made you happy during the day (the sunrise, a child's laughter, something that went your way) and write them down in a happiness journal.
5. Practice Positive EFT. Up next.

"We have to teach our clients to focus on the good in their lives. Admittedly, for folks with a history of trauma, they have created deep neurological grooves and are very good at focusing on the junk, noticing how bad they feel, noticing what's not right in their lives or in the world, etc.

"I once had a hypnosis teacher named Stephen Parkhill. He was good at regressing folks back to the root cause issues underlying physical and emotional diseases and clearing out the traumas. After doing this work for 20 years with thousands of clients, he made the comment, 'No matter how much manure (trauma) you shovel out of the stall, the clients won't get better and stay that way until they learn to focus on the good in their lives.' The point is, healing is not just about clearing away trauma. It's about learning to feel good, learning to handle increased energy flow."

~ ERIC. B. ROBINS, M.D.

Positive EFT

I often end a client session with this gentle yet powerful energy exercise that I learned in Positive EFT by Silvia Hartmann:

Choose something you really want in your life.

Put both hands on your chest in the Heart Position, take three deep breaths and say the name of the positive energy out aloud. Then lightly tap all of the special energy points, starting from the top of the head. On each point, say the name of the positive energy loudly and clearly as you tap. Take a deep breath in and out, then move on to the next point. Finish in the Heart Position and take three deep breaths.[6]

---

6 Reproduced with permission from Silvia Hartmann, Director of the Guild of Energists; developer and primary designer of Energy EFT, Positive EFT, Project Sanctuary, The Genius Symbols, EMO Energy In Motion, Events Psychology and Modern Stress Management.

Positive EFT as a Meditation

And here is my own spin on this lovely exercise which I now use as a form of meditation while lying in bed before falling asleep at night and (often) in the morning on waking up:

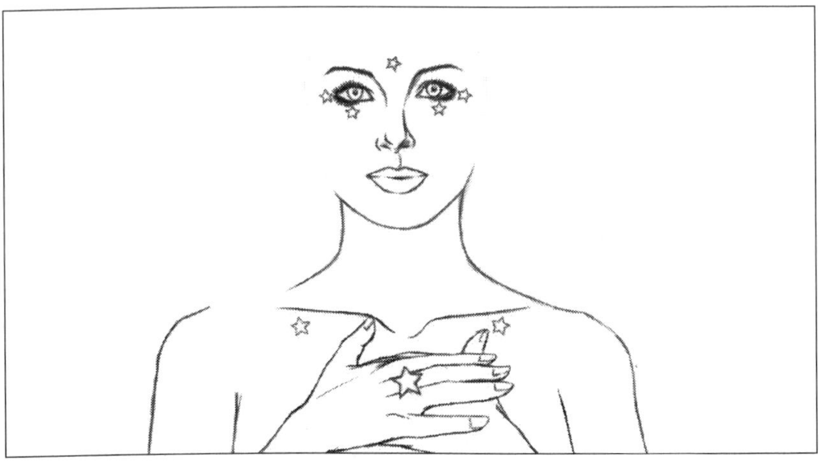

Positive EFT Tapping Points

1. Select a positive word or phrase such as "love," "calm," or "peace"... any desired feeling or state of mind that you want for yourself.

2. Focus on breathing slowly, deeply, and peacefully.

3. With both hands on your chest in the Heart Position, take a deep, calm breath, say or mentally embrace the word, and exhale. Repeat twice.

4. Touch the energy points in turn, breathing in, saying or thinking the positive word, and exhaling.

5. Finish with three deep breaths in the Heart Position.

This is the exercise that has allowed me to sleep deeply, after decades of attempting other methods to cure insomnia that had plagued me since childhood.

I would be very interested to hear how this method works for you. Direct your message to mia@miadoucet.com and I promise to respond.

Clients Who Have Transformed Their World

My work is 100% confidential.
But some of my clients graciously allow me to share their results.

Three current "Transformation" clients wanted their comments included in these pages.

(One of them insisted.)

I am grateful to them ...

"When I came to you I felt void of emotion and passion, like I was hollow. Our first five sessions changed the trajectory of my life. Tapping reopened my soul by quickly clearing out old wounds that I had carried with me for the majority of my life. I find I'm so much more of me now, much more honest, much more comfortable in my own skin. I don't hate myself for things that weren't my fault. I can talk about stuff like I was raped when I was seven without falling apart. I used to beat myself up for so many life choices I viewed as poor. I've been able to clear those feelings through Tapping and recognize the past for what it is - the PAST. Living in the present, I can be anything and everything I want to be—other than a singer, because all the lessons and tapping in the world would not put me on The Voice!"

~ Heather White, Vice-President, Sales & Marketing

"I'm a believer! It's been transformational. Eight years of talk therapy got me nowhere except it was a good place to complain. Your style is great toward getting to the issues and getting them resolved. Childhood traumas and negativity that have been hanging over me for my whole life are gone. The anger is gone. This is the most peaceful my life has ever been. I feel good. I feel free, for the first time ever. I'm a different person. I finally value myself. The track

I was on was killing me but now I have the confidence to finally step back and make positive changes in my life. Because I matter."

~ Kim Petry, CPA, Chief Financial Officer

"If you are willing to put your skepticism aside and go into the deep dark corners of your soul, tapping will truly transform your life. I highly recommend working with Mia Doucet. She has awoken an empowerment within me to create a life I only dreamed possible."

~ Jane Rusciolelli, Educator

Glossary

Glossary

Ask & Receive

Ask & Receive is an exciting new health discovery that uses the power of your unlimited being to allow you to ask for what you want in your life and have it! People are using this simple process to ask for changes in every part of their lives; greater health, less pain, releasing trauma, more joy, greater flexibility, better relationships, peace. People are asking for and receiving all of these things and many more.

Ask and Receive understands that our early traumas and resulting limiting beliefs form the background of all future experience. When our unlimited being is able to quickly release these limitations we are left feeling happier, healthier and more in alignment with our higher purpose.

Source: http://askandreceive.org

EFT (Emotional Freedom Techniques)

EFT is a meridian-based healing modality "based on the same principles that have been used for thousands of years in acupuncture—but without the needles." EFT is a powerful process for eliminating phobias, traumatic memories including Post-

Traumatic Stress Disorder (PTSD), addictive cravings, depression, anxieties, panic attacks, physical ailments, worry, anger, guilt, grief and all the other limiting emotions that inhibit one's personal happiness and performance in business, sports and the arts.

Founded by Gary Craig in 1995, EFT rapidly spread into a worldwide phenomenon. Today, EFT is often combined with other methods and refers to a wide variety of different tapping techniques.

Writes Gary Craig: "However, this wide variety of 'things called EFT' causes confusion for the public, and it has become very challenging for newcomers to distinguish the original, actual EFT from all the variations. Accordingly, I have established a new trademarked term, **Official EFT™** that only includes the true EFT instruction as I have created and refined it."

Source: http://www.emofree.com

FASTEREFT (FASTER EMOTIONALLY FOCUSED TRANSFORMATIONS)

FasterEFT is a methodology developed by Robert G. Smith. It is a collection of cutting-edge techniques and processes that integrate into one system the best and most effective elements of EFT (Emotional Freedom Techniques), BSFF (Be Set Free Fast), NLP (Neuro-Linguistic Programming), Matrix Reimprinting, spiritual understanding, and the latest scientific discoveries of the mind's great ability to heal and transform a person's life.

"FasterEFT addresses the entire mind/body system which includes what you think and how you process your thoughts, along with the body's response. It is a self-empowering system that gives you control over your past, present and your future. It will show you how to design and transform your life right now."

Source: http://fastereft.com

There has been much discussion in the tapping community about some of the latest FasterEFT practices. The feeling is that some of these methods are too provocative and may unnecessarily re-traumatize clients. The organization, at the time of this writing, has been working on solidifying a code of ethics, as well as instituting safety training for the practitioners so that they work within their scope of practice.

MATRIX REIMPRINTING

Matrix Reimprinting, by Karl Dawson, evolved from and builds upon EFT. It is a method for transforming a negative memory once the painful emotional charge associated with the memory has been resolved through tapping.

The method involves going back into the memory and changing the way our mind has encoded the experience. Rewriting memories changes our personal history through providing our younger self with positive resources such as love, safety, perspective, personal strength, and confidence that were not available to us at the time of the painful event.

MERIDIANS

The meridian system is a complex network of invisible energy pathways that interconnect throughout the entire body. We tap on the meridian points that are easily accessible on the surface of the body.

All three emotional freedom energy modalities above involve tapping on the meridian system.

NLP (Neuro-Linguistic Programming)

The technology of Neuro-linguistic Programming was co-created and co-founded by Richard Bandler and John Grinder in the 1970's. In simple terms, NLP is the study of how we think, how we structure our thoughts, how we communicate, and how we internally process our experiences. Its ultimate goal is to change the past and the future through restructuring our thinking in the present.

NLP codified the work of three illustrious therapists: Dr. Milton H. Erickson, Virginia Satir and Fritz Perls.

In one way or another, NLP's combination of techniques as had a profound influence not just on therapeutic disciplines, but on sports, corporate management training, team building, teaching, coaching, and sales and negotiation strategies.

NLP is a component of many energy practices.

Positive EFT

Silvia Hartmann, Founder of Positive EFT, discovered that when we work with positive energies exclusively and in the correct way, there is no need to tap on the past. "(Positive EFT) has become a fine tool to create and sculpt the future you want, increases confidence and makes you excited about what comes next in your life."

TENSION & TRAUMA RELEASING EXERCISES (TRE)

Tension & Trauma Release Exercises (TRE), are a set of simple body stretches and movements, developed by Dr. David Berceli. They are designed to activate an autonomic tremor mechanism in the body. These 'neurogenic' tremors appear to travel through the body with the assistance of Central Pattern Generators in the spinal column. Repeated activation of this tremor mechanism seems to relax physical tension patterns in the body that are the result of past stressful experiences. The resulting effect appears to calm down the central nervous system by releasing these areas of chronic tension from the musculature. By continuously activating this tremor mechanism, a reorganizational behavior seems to emerge in the individual's brain, spine, nervous & myofascial systems, as well as their life as a whole.

For more information about this process go to:
www.traumaprevention.com.

Source: Dr. David Berceli

THOUGHT FIELD THERAPY (TFT)

Thought Field Therapy (TFT) was the brainchild of the late Dr. Roger Callahan. A psychologist, he broke with traditional psychotherapy to combine Applied Kinesiology and acupuncture to treat patients.

Dr. Callahan discovered Causal Diagnosis – a way to find and eliminate negative emotions at source – and maintained that there was a certain (and elaborate) algorithm for treating different problems.

Gary Craig paid $110,000 for the original Callaghan Techniques® and Voice Technology™ training. He then simplified the tapping system, and eliminated the need for algorithms to diagnose which meridians to tap in sequence for specific emotions, and made EFT available to the layperson at a nominal fee.

Dr. Callahan was most proud of his discovery of Psychological Reversal, which he claimed is what blocks treatments from working.

Some have called into question lately the idea of Psychological Reversal. Perhaps it depends how you define the term. I think of it as a deep, hidden (and therefore unconscious) conflict that causes a person to act in ways that contradict a stated goal. That would help explain the resistance, avoidance, procrastination and other self-sabotaging behaviors we so often experience.

Without Roger Callahan's groundbreaking discoveries, none of today's simplified meridian tapping techniques would exist.

Trance

Trance is a naturally occurring, altered state of consciousness.

For most people, trance occurs naturally and frequently throughout the day. The more obvious trances are daydreams, emotional involvement in a movie or television program, and the state most of us are in when driving or engaged in a well-rehearsed activity.

Any time that we go back to a past memory in our mind's eye (whether that memory be an internal movie, a feeling, a sound, a smell, or a body sensation) and we are not consciously aware in the present moment, we are in a state of trance.

Resources

Church, Dawson. *The Genie in Your Genes: Epigenetic Medicine and the New Biology of Intention.* Fulton, California: Energy Psychology Press, 2014 (3rd Edition)

Dawson, Karl and Marillat, Kate. *Transform Your Beliefs, Transform Your Life: EFT Tapping Using Matrix Reimprinting.* Hay House UK, 2014

Feinstein, David, Eden, Donna, and Craig, Gary. *The Promise of Energy Psychology: Revolutionary Tools for Dramatic Personal Change.* NY: Jeremy P. Tarcher/The Penguin Group, 2005

Lipton, Bruce H. Ph.D. Ph.D. *The Biology of Belief 10th Anniversary Edition: Unleashing the Power of Consciousness, Matter & Miracles.* Carlsbad, California: Hay House, Inc., 2016

Ortner, Nick. *The Tapping Solution: A Revolutionary System for Stress-Free Living.* Carlsbad, California: Hay House, Inc., 2013

Wells, Steve. *100% YES! The Energy of Success: Release Your Resistance Align Your Values Go for Your Goals Using Simple Energy Techniques (SET).* Western Australia: Waterford Publishing, 2016

About the Author

Mia Doucet has always been fascinated by what makes people tick. Since university graduation she's had one foot in the business world and one foot in the world of energy psychology. This book signals that the latter has finally won out.

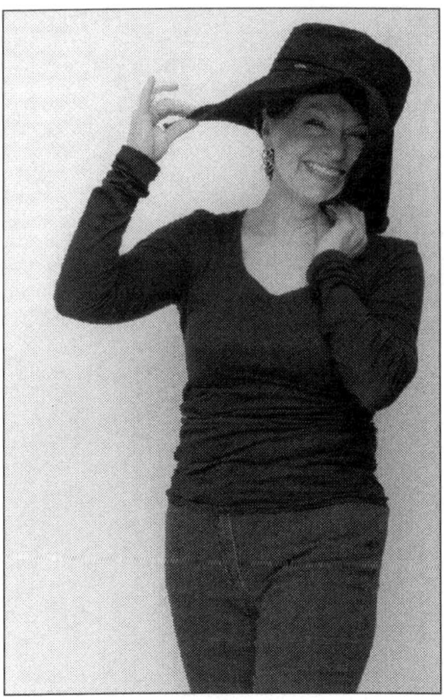

After a career in education, manufacturing and banking, corporate training, and consulting with Fortune 100 and Fortune 500 manufacturing firms Mia has chosen to focus full-time on helping people transform their lives. She serves a global clientele.

Mia holds a degree in education. In addition to having studied various disciplines including Gestalt Therapy, One Brain®, NLP, Meridian Tapping and Awakening Dynamics, she has professional certifications in coaching, sales, consulting, and human resources and is an award winning author.

Mia's specialty is working with the tougher cases … people who have "tried everything" and not had the promised results.

Her strengths as a practitioner include strong intuition, the ability to identify core patterns and subconscious programs, and the skill to clear them quickly, easily and painlessly.

Mia Doucet offers customized, one on one sessions to people who are committed to transforming their lives and who don't want to have to spend the $100,000 ++ it cost her to get to a happy state.

She welcomes you to contact her directly:

Direct Email: mia@miadoucet.com

Website: http://TAPPINGTransformYourWorld/contact

Website: http://miadoucet.com/contact

LinkedIn: www.linkedin.com/in/miadoucet/

Facebook: TAPPING | Transform Your World

ALSO BY MIA DOUCET

ENERGY PSYCHOLOGY

FIBROMYALGIA: Secrets of a Fibro Survivor

BUSINESS

CHINA IN MOTION | 17 Secrets to Slashing the Time to Production, to Market, and to Profits in China, Japan and South Korea

REVEALED: 7 Reasons Why Your Teams Underperform And How To Fix Them

BUSINESS (KINDLE)

CHINA BUSINESS SECRETS:
Give Face or Get Lost
Pray to the Right Buddha
Keep It Serious and Social
Wipe That Expression Off Your Face
Leave Western Ways At Home
Protect Tiger Lured from Mountains

INVITATION TO POST A REVIEW

Thank you for reading!

If you enjoyed this book and feel it would be of value to others, would you consider letting others know about it by writing a review?

I ask because, as a reader, you have the power to make the information available to more people with your comments on Amazon.

If you like the idea, I will send you a quick, easy little one-page-how-to that will make it a snap.

If you disagree with what I have written, or if you didn't enjoy the book, I would also like to hear from you.

Either way, you can reach me directly by email: mia@miadoucet.com or via my website: www.TappingTransformYourWorld.com/contact.

To ensure that I can identify your email message if it gets caught in my finicky Outlook filters, write *About Your Book* in the Subject line.

All the best,
Mia

ENDNOTES

i http://miadoucet.com | http://speedtoroi.global/

ii FIBROMYALGIA: Secrets of a Fibro Survivor https://www.amazon.com

iii If you want more information on fractals, you will find it on the Fractal Foundation website, http://fractalfoundation.org.

iv Fedor Andreev, Ph.D., Professor of Mathematical Physics, Western Illinois University

v Photo downloaded from Flickr: https:www.flickr.com/photos/mararie by Creative Commons licensing.

vi This video was shot years ago. I no longer find it useful to tap under the arm or breast.

vii Excerpted from the book Money and the Law of Attraction by Esther and Jerry Hicks, Hay House, 2008, California

viii Matrix Reimprinting is a ground-breaking therapy that focuses on connecting with our child self to transform core beliefs that not only control our lives but actually create events in our lives.

ix In late August 2013, Psychological Science released the results of a 16-year, first-of-its-kind study of 1,420 participants titled "Impact of Bullying in Childhood on Adult Health, Wealth, Crime, and Social Outcomes." The article is available if you want to read the details. http://journals.sagepub.com/search/advanced

x See above reference to the study on bullying as reported in Psychological Science, August 19, 2013.

xi The Holographic Universe. The article refers to the work of Karl H. Pribram (1919-2015), Neurosurgeon, Neuroscientist, Professor (Yale, Stanford Universities), "recipient of more than sixty major international awards and honors."

xii Steve Wells, *100% YES! The Energy of Success: Release Your Resistance Align Your Values Go for Your Goals Using Simple Energy Techniques (SET)* (Western Australia: Waterford Publishing, 2016)

xiii http://fractalfoundation.org

76287339R00133

Made in the USA
Columbia, SC
04 September 2017